FIGHTING CANCER

with the — THALI

Rita Date
Dr. Seema Sonis

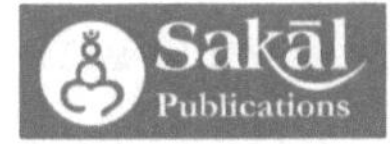

Sakāl Publications

Fighting Cancer with the Thali

Sakal Media Pvt. Ltd.
595, Budhwar Peth,
Pune – 411002, India

www.sakalpublications.com
sakalprakashan@esakal.com

First Edition: December 2023

ISBN No.: 978-81-19311-41-5

Edited by: Niyati Joshi
Cover Design: Pallavi Chidrawar Vyawahare
Typesetting: Gouri Kharade

Printed in India by Sakal Media Pvt. Ltd.

*This book is dedicated to
All those who have experienced cancer,
Given care to cancer patients, or
Suffered the loss of a loved one due to this disease.
May this book offer support, understanding, and
inspiration on your path to healing.*

Table of Contents

Foreword

"One-fourth of what you eat keep you alive. Three-fourth of what you eat keep your doctor alive."

- Dr. Andrew Sauls

We need to eat so little to survive, yet we eat so much that we suffer from various lifestyle diseases that only feed the healthcare industry, which is one of the world's most profiteering, multi-billion-dollar industries today.

Improper and excessive diet and the lack of exercise are the root causes of disease. The increasing burden of lifestyle diseases such as cancer, heart issues, diabetes, and arthritis are solely caused by indiscretions in diet and sedentary habits.

Rita Date has been part of the Prashanti Cancer Care team for many years. She gives valuable advice on nutrition to patients, and I am happy that patients from all over India will now have this book as a resource during their treatment. There are very few books that impart nutrition advice for cancer patients, specifically for the Indian population. The authors have also clearly and beautifully laid down the changing scenario of diet and disease in our country. The incidence of cancer in India was low compared to the western world, but today, we are catching up with the western world in every respect relating to lifestyle and disease.

The concept of the thali is the essence of our culinary culture, and unfortunately, it is not one to which we give much thought. It is, in fact, nutritionally sound and a major contributor to a healthy lifestyle. This thali was properly thought out and laid down by our ancestors. **Rita and her co-author Seema have beautifully epitomized and made the thali central to the concept of healthy living, giving insight into describing and formulating a healthy diet based on the traditional Thali.** The book provides easy reading into some fundamental causes of disease and explains the basis of disease prevention with a healthy lifestyle.

The authors have made a commendable effort to address various aspects of situations demanding changes in diet plans with recommendations and solutions for the same. The book would be a handy guide to care givers and patients during chemotherapy and help them understand the steps to improve immunity and combat stressful situations during and after cancer treatment. Fatigue post-treatment is a formidable side effect of cancer treatment; only careful planning of one's diet and exercise regimes can help to overcome it. This has been nicely alluded to in the book. Obesity is another problem that affects cancer patients immediately post-chemotherapy. This needs to be avoided to ensure better cure rates and can only be done with strict adherence to a diet and exercise protocol. This again is addressed with clarity and credible advice.

"*Fighting Cancer with the Thali*" systematically takes one through all diet-related information during and after cancer and is a must-read for cancer patients and their caregivers.

Dr. Chaitanand Koppikar

(Dr. Koppikar is a Consulting Oncosurgeon, Ruby Hall, Jehangir Hospital, Pune and Hinduja Healthcare Surgical, Mumbai, Founding Medical Director and Managing Trustee, Prashanti Cancer Care Mission, Pune and Founder, Centre for Translational Cancer Research, Pune.)

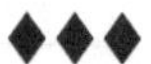

Introduction

Rita Date

If you have picked up this book, chances are that you or someone close to you is going through a difficult time with cancer. A cancer diagnosis is shocking and scary. The internet is filled with advice and information, much of it conflicting. But it is an irrefutable fact that the disease of cancer is spreading, and we need to know how best to combat it.

I was on my annual trip to Boston to visit my parents when my son Nishant's (Nishu) illness started with a fever. The next day, a rash erupted, and on the day after that came chilling pains across his bones and muscles. Diarrhea began soon after. The pediatrician told us it was a viral flu, but after a week of only giving Tylenol, the symptoms were only getting worse, and then the same doctor told us to take him to Children's Hospital in Boston. He was admitted, and then a battery of tests began. Specialists from all fields came to see him – dermatologists, infectious disease doctors (since we were visiting from India), rheumatologists, nephrologists, GPs, and oncologists. No one could figure out what was wrong.

After being intensely pricked and prodded, Nishu had no usable veins left in his arm, so the area around his feet had to be tapped for blood. Repeated diarrhea had left his anal area raw and bruised. But CT scans, MRIs, and biopsies did not reveal anything wrong, and no diagnosis was given even after a week in the hospital. Then his blood count dropped, and he needed a transfusion. Until that point, the doctors said all his organs were working adequately, but suddenly, he needed help breathing. He was intubated and taken to the ICU.

Two days later, a doctor rushed into the waiting room and told my husband and me that Nishu's heart was failing, and he needed to be put on an ECMO (extracorporeal membrane oxygenation machine) to help support it. An ECMO basically does the work of the heart and lungs for the patient. It is usually used as a last resort.

Special tubes called cannulas were put into his blood vessels. These cannulas used a pump to transfer the blood from his heart and push it through tubes to a machine where it received oxygen and removed its carbon dioxide. Next, the blood was warmed to body temperature and sent back into Nishu's body through another cannula. There was a 40% survival rate for this procedure. So much could have gone wrong, but Nishu pulled through and successfully came off the machine one week later.

Finally, he was diagnosed with HLH – hemophagocytic lymphohistiosis – a rare disease that attacks all organs. Eight weeks of chemo began soon after and Nishu slowly got better. However, in the last week of chemo, he had a relapse in the form of meningitis and was required to stay in the hospital for an additional 6 weeks. We were told that the only course of treatment would be a bone marrow transplant. Another round of tests and repeated chemo were required to get him ready for the transplant. Luckily, my daughter, Saya, who was only ten at the time, was able to be his marrow donor. She was brave and did her part to save her brother.

He remained in the hospital for nearly two months after the transplant. Watching your child suffer such pain is heartbreaking; you wish you could take their place. Children often don't remember the time spent in a hospital, but parents never forget it. After the transplant, we celebrated every milestone: one month, three months, six months! Luck was on our side, and Nishu did not suffer too many of the lasting side effects of the transplant.

Throughout this harrowing time, Nishu's diet was top priority for us. Family and friends in the US and India banded together to help us through this ordeal. My mother-in-law flew in from India, and she and my mother made fresh, home-cooked meals for Nishu every day. Along with chemo, the steroids that were part of his protocol turned out to be a blessing. Steroids increased his appetite, and he ate well. He only wanted Indian vegetarian food and only certain *sabjis*. Nishu's favorite veggies were *tondli*, *bhindi*, and *methi*. Not easily available in Boston winters, my mother would make frequent trips to the Indian store to procure them. My mother made *idlis* and a variety of *dosas* for breakfast every morning. Both she and my mother-in-law made *chapatis*, *sabjis*, dal, rice, and *dahi* for lunch and dinner. A considerable amount of time and effort was placed into making these meals. Luckily, Nishu savored every bite of his *thali*. It was a delight to watch him eat.

He craved no sweets, and just the sight of any other types of food he used to love – chicken, fish, Chinese, *chaat*, burgers, pizza, and pasta – would make him lose his appetite. Even when Saya urged him to eat a slice of pizza, he refused. He only wanted his roti-sabji-dal-chawal, and a meal was never complete without his *dahi*.

Many factors contributed to Nishu's recovery, and not all were in our control. Nutrition, though, was something we could influence and manage, which proved to be a big factor in his recovery. The right nutrition gave him the strength to fight his disease and mitigate the unwanted consequences of the harmful drugs needed to fight it. This experience was the reason I started to champion the cause of eating homemade food for better health. Working as a nutritionist in a cancer clinic, I realized that many cancer patients needed help knowing what to eat during treatment. I knew a book was needed, and I recruited

Seema Sonis, my good friend and medico-dietician, to be my partner in this endeavor.

We finished the final manuscript of this book in February of 2020, but Covid hit the world, and cancer took a backseat. Unfortunately, cancer cases continued to rise in our country during this period. India is fortunate to have certain ancient tools that are beneficial to fight the disease, both in preventing and mitigating side effects of the treatment protocols. Yoga, pranayama, meditation, and homemade food are part of our cultural landscape. It is time we return to these practices to help us live healthier to combat cancer and other lifestyle diseases.

Illnesses like cancer can make people feel like they have lost control over their lives. There is, however, an important aspect of health you can always control, and that is the nourishment you put in your body. Common everyday foods can be used to assist the healing process. It is unnecessary to spend money on fancy foreign foods you've read about or that some friend insists will cure your cancer. Only the treatment your oncologist prescribes can treat your cancer, but nutrition will strengthen your body to fight the disease and help you recuperate after the treatment.

Cancer is the most unpredictable and complex of all non-communicable diseases and has emerged as a major threat and cause of global mortality. The World Health Organization (WHO) has estimated that a staggering 35% of cancers worldwide are caused by diet. A substantial rise in obesity rates has also contributed to various diseases such as diabetes and heart disease. Cancer, too, is one of the consequences of obesity. Better food quality and eating habits are much-needed ways to prevent diseases.

Several books have been published that address nutrition and cancer, but few target the specific needs of the Indian population. This book emphasizes upon the wisdom of India's rich food heritage and its most widely available healing foods. Healing foods are those that prevent cancer as well as help overcome it.

The following pages will address:

- What to eat in order to help prevent cancer
- What to eat in order to boost your ability to deal with side-effects when undergoing cancer treatment
- What to eat after treatment in order to thrive, not just survive
- A prescription on how to be healthy in mind, body, and spirit through the MNM Principle

Every part of our nation has some form of a 'thali' or plate on which a meal is served. Today, the word 'thali' has evolved to mean a complete meal for one at a restaurant served on a large platter filled with several food items served in small *katoris* (bowls). This is to distinguish it from the a la carte menu option of ordering *sabji, dal, roti* (vegetable, dal, bread) and rice individually, which you serve yourself on your plate. The traditional *thali* contains a balance of carbohydrates, protein, fats, vitamins and minerals needed to supply the energy required to live a healthy life. A restaurant meal is not the *thali* we are advocating. Whether it is a 5-star restaurant or a local canteen *thali*, it can in no way be compared to one that's been home-cooked. Real food cooked at home is needed to win the war against cancer.

In order to fight the growing burden of cancer and improve health, even our homemade *thalis* need improvement. Proportions of vegetables to grains need to be skewed to better suit the world we are currently living in. For example, as a rule, we do not move around as much as our grandparents or parents once did; they walked or cycled everywhere and did not sit for hours working on laptops. Therefore, we cannot burn the amount of carbohydrates and fats incorporated in the traditional *thali*, which was created to meet very different nutritional needs. Additionally, we are not eating enough fresh vegetables. Even if you are not a vegetarian, your plate should still be filled with fifty percent vegetables.

This book is full of positivity. Our goal is to remind people of India's wonderful food heritage and the healing power it possesses. Hippocrates gets credit for the phrase "let food be thy medicine," but Ayurveda, the science of using food as medicine, is 5,000 years old, pre-dating the works of Greek philosophers and scientists.

Ayurveda is a science based on the premise that most diseases originate in the stomach; our ancestors knew the importance of the 'gut' well before it became a buzzword. Reading the *shlokas* (verses) of ancient Ayurvedic texts brings a sense of pride. Civilization in the Indus valley understood the importance of food, movement, and mind – concepts that are relevant today and can be relearned by going back to our roots.

Over the past decade, the study of nutrition has expanded, and the general public understands the impact of food on preventing cancer better. After several years of investigating findings from our own practices, we have undertaken to write this book.

In India we have age old wisdom on how to live healthy lives. We hope this book helps you to find this wisdom helpful in your cancer journey, whether it be prevention or treatment support.

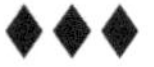

कोऽरुक कोऽरुक?
हितभूक् मित्तभूक् सोऽरुक् सोऽरुक्।

चरकसंहिता

Charkacharya asks
"Tell me, who is healthy?"
He himself answers
"One who eats less,
one who eats the right food is healthy."

Charak Samhita

MNM – The Mind-Nutrition Movement Principle

According to traditional medicine, the mind, body, and soul have been segregated. Modern medicine focuses on the body, ignoring the mind and creating a purely mechanical view of treating illness. Bodies are seen as machines to be fixed with the available tools, not as souls that need to be healed. This is a Western view of medicine, and it also dominates healthcare in India. But this has not always been the case. In India, we have always had healthy diets, a strong sense of spirituality, and a vibrant network of close family. Our ancient traditions of Ayurveda, yoga, and pranayama were somehow always integrated into our daily life. Think back to school when prayers, rituals, and yoga were part of Physical Education.

There are no absolutes or guarantees when it comes to developing cancer. Although science has proven that cancer develops through unhealthy cell reproduction, we do not always know why. We know that fifty percent of cancers come from lifestyle factors – diet, smoking, and chewing tobacco being the biggest culprits. Although not every person who smokes or is obese will get cancer, their chances of getting it are much higher than someone who maintains a healthy lifestyle and does not smoke. In other words, fifty percent of cancer prevention is within our control, and we should take every advantage of this fact.

Since the advent of widespread industrialization in the early 1990s, the nation's health has deteriorated, made evident by heart disease, diabetes, obesity, and cancers that have increased significantly. Why is it so difficult to stay healthy? The open economy and competition have raised millions of Indians into middle class, but the road to get there was full of traps. Fast food and sedentary lifestyles became the norm. Long working hours and long commute times meant no energy at the end of the day and no time to cook. Eating out seemed to be a necessary part of the new working culture. Fewer home-cooked meals and more restaurant food and fast food accompanied by drinking and smoking resulted in a rise in obesity and disease. Companies took note and added wellness programs and health check-ups, but these measures did not tackle the root causes of deteriorating health due to ongoing work stress and home issues, coupled with junk food and sedentary lifestyles.

> *In her book, Radical Remission, author Kelly Turner, Ph.D., analyzed more than 1000 cases of statistically unexpected cancer remission. She found nine elements that were present in almost every case. These were:*
>
> 1. *A radical change in diet*
> 2. *Taking control of health*
> 3. *Following intuition*
> 4. *Using herbs and supplements*
> 5. *Releasing suppressed emotions*
> 6. *Embracing social support*
> 7. *Increasing positive emotions*
> 8. *Deepening spiritual connection*
> 9. *Having a strong reason for living*

This book focuses on nutrition, but the mind-body connection cannot be overlooked as it is integral to one's health and healing. For example, your state of mind while cooking or eating can influence the effect food has on your body. Thoughts that focus on losing control, financial insecurities, and fear of death are natural after getting a cancer diagnosis, but too many pessimistic thoughts can have an unfavorable impact on your recovery.

MNM stands for three words: Mind, Nutrition, and Movement. It is the template for healthy living that we give to our patients. It sounds simple, but if it were, we would not be facing rising rates of disease in India.

Simple steps can lead to profound change.

Chapter 1

Mind Over Cancer

Yanira Daes, the owner of Soham Yoga Studio in West Palm Beach, Florida is 53 years old but doesn't look a day over 40. I (Rita) took a few yoga classes with her and learned her fascinating story. Yani was diagnosed with breast cancer in 2012, and a lumpectomy and mastectomy soon followed. Yanira decided to fight her cancer by drastically changing her diet. She eliminated all meat and dairy and began eating plenty of fresh fruits, vegetables, sprouts, and dals, even learning to cook Indian dal, *khichdi*, and lentils. Giving up meat didn't come easy since Yanira is originally from Venezuela, where beef is a staple on the plate. What impressed me the most was Yanira's entry into yoga, which she began learning right after her diagnosis, starting with pranayama to bring more oxygen and energy into her body. Soon after, she began with some easy asanas (after getting the go-ahead from her doctor). She was in pain during the poses but was determined to get stronger, so she set a goal for herself and worked towards achieving it. In 2015, only three years after her diagnosis, Yanira, now completely in remission, completed teacher training in Ashtanga yoga, a physically demanding type of yoga. And soon after that, she opened her own yoga studio, where she now teaches many forms of yoga. Yanira believes that positivity and sheer determination helped her with her recovery.

Although all three elements in our MNM principle are important to maintain a healthy life, one's state of mind and attitude perhaps play the most important role. Eating well and getting the exercise you need are no doubt essential. However, having the right frame of mind is crucial and can immensely impact your health. Countless stories like Yanira's concerning mind over matter in combating disease abound; a strong and well-balanced mind can overcome many of life's obstacles and stresses.

Stress and anxiety can cause a multitude of health problems. Some short-term stress is good for the body, but when it becomes chronic, the body responds negatively. Everyone has some difficult demands in their lives, but how we control its effect on us determines how it affects our bodies. The right practices to help with managing stress and anxiety are essential for a healthy lifestyle.

Stress can manifest itself in many ways in the body. Heart trouble, inability to sleep, acidity, weight loss, weight gain, and yeast infections are among a long list of health problems it can cause.

Cortisol is a stress hormone, and high cortisol levels interfere with learning, memory, immune function, bone density, blood pressure, and much more. Cortisol is released in response to fear or stress by the adrenal glands as part of the fight-or-flight response. This primal survival mechanism enabled ancient humans and other mammals to react quickly to life-threatening situations by fighting the threat or fleeing to safety. These days, we are no longer running from lions and tigers, but unfortunately, the body's cortisol response is triggered by non-life-threatening stressors such as traffic jams, work pressure, and family issues.

Several studies show a relationship between stress and cancer. In our practices, we have seen the impact the mind has on the healing and recovery of disease, especially cancer. Your attitude plays perhaps the most important role in whether you just survive or thrive after cancer treatment.

Our minds, emotions, and cognitive behavioral factors affect our physiology and biochemistry. This scientifically proven fact is an important part of cancer treatment, especially since biochemistry determines how the body will respond to the cancer attack. For example, studies show that news of a cancer diagnosis itself has a profound negative effect on a person's health. The mental-emotional connection to human physiology and treatment protocols has been proven time and again by science. Psychological stressors, for instance, are known to have a significant impact on your body's immune response and on every cell in the body.

Research indicates that simple daily relaxation practices can produce changes in gene expression that may help in inhibiting specific cancer-promotion factors, curb inflammation, and counter malignant growth. All this enhances cancer treatment.

Yoga has proved time after time to reduce stress and anxiety. Yoga reduces cortisol levels in the body. All limbs of yoga – asanas (postures), pranayama (deep breathing techniques), and dhyana (meditation) have individually proven to bring down cortisol.

Just as we nourish the body with healthy food, we must also nourish the soul. Some stress relief tools, such as exercising, eating healthy, and having a social network, are tangible. A less tangible but no less useful way to fight stress is through spirituality. Feeling whole and fulfilled spiritually plays an important healing role.

Whether it's organized religion in a church, temple, mosque, or an individual path of meditation and contemplation, some form of spirituality is necessary to keep us grounded.

Yoga

"Yoga Chitta Vritti Nirodhah"
(Yoga is stilling the fluctuations of the mind)

– Lord Patanjali

Mind, we maintain, is the most important element of the MNM principle. Yoga removes impurities from various levels of the mind and unites the body and mind with the spirit. It also trains the body and mind to self-observe and helps us become aware of our own nature. Yoga's purpose is to cultivate discernment, awareness, self-regulation, and higher consciousness in the individual.

Yoga promotes physical relaxation by decreasing the activity of the sympathetic nervous system, which lowers the heart rate and increases breath volume. The sympathetic nervous system is the part of the autonomic nervous system that prepares the body to react to stresses such as threat or injury.

Yoga is the need of the day and should be integrated into our daily life. Numerous studies have shown that yoga practices have played a significant role in reducing stress levels. Stress causes many responses in the body, leading to a variety of ailments, including cancer. Entire books have been written on how the various limbs of yoga can help play a significant role in maintaining good health.

Yoga works specifically in two ways: physically or externally and spiritually or internally. Asanas are a small but necessary part of this practice. Asanas energize the body while calming the mind and preparing the body for deeper meditation. The elation you feel after doing asanas is different from the high you get from running, cycling, or going to the gym. However, these physical benefits are not their purpose. Yoga is meant to resolve the blocking and distortion of the mind that keep you from knowing yourself. The physical aspect of yoga is an added benefit.

Lord Patanjali, the author of the Yoga Sutras was aware of the mind-body connection and the role asanas play in preparing the body before embarking on the quest of unification of the mind, body, and spirit. His definition of Yoga is the removing of the fluctuations of the mind. In other words, the practice of yoga helps still the mind until it rests in a state of total and utter tranquility so that one can experience life as it is.

Pranayama

When we feel fearful, we hold our breath or take shallow and uneven breaths. Pranayama, which combines *prana* (breath), with *yama* (extension or control) is the formal practice of controlling the breath and plays a vital role in yoga. Bringing attention to the rhythm of your breath can do wonders for your stress levels and enable oxygen to move freely through the body. Pranayama includes various breathing techniques such as abdominal breathing and alternate-nostril breathing, opening up the chest for the smooth passage of breath. Through pranayama, one learns to breathe slowly and deeply in rhythmic patterns that strengthen the respiratory system and calm the nervous system. If performed properly, these practices can dissolve stress and emotional distress, freeing the mind from anxiety.

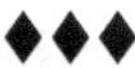

Modern Diet and Cancer

Nutrition

*"Eating does not mean merely filling up the stomach
to satisfy hunger, rather it is Yadna-karma."*

- Indian sages

There are two dangers when it comes to nutrition science. The first is to focus too much on it. Several clients have come to the authors with questions about certain miracle foods they read about online and think it will prevent or reverse their disease. Even the best nutritional practices cannot completely reverse the damage already done to the body by disease. Years of poor eating habits will take even more years of eating optimally for any reversal to begin. However, it is better to start late than never to eat healthy. And please note, there are no miracle foods that can reverse this disease.

The second danger of nutrition, and perhaps the more perilous of the two, is to think too little of it. The primary focus of this book is the importance of what you eat and how this can impact the body before, during, and after cancer treatment. And there's a reason for this: both authors have seen the profound effect nutrition has on disease development. Moreover, global nutrition studies have proven the ways the type of food we eat impacts our response to disease. Large-scale clinical trials have shown that nutrients found in foods are necessary for healing and should be included in treatment plans.

How we nurture our bodies is crucial to living a healthy life. We need nutrients consistently, otherwise deficiencies develop. When nutrient deficiencies go unaddressed, diseases may occur, as the body does not have adequate tools to fight them.

> *Obesity will become chief cause of cancer in few decades*
>
> *Research published in the British Journal of cancer shows that obesity can be the risk factor for 13 different types of cancer, including colon, breast, kidney, and uterine cancers. The world's largest independent cancer research body pointed out that obesity could overtake smoking in the coming year as the main avoidable cause of cancer related deaths (Arnold, M. et al, 2016).*

For example, several studies show that women whose diet is high in fruits, vegetables, and pulses and minimize red meat, salt, and processed carbohydrates lower their chances of getting estrogen **receptor positive** breast cancer, which accounts for a quarter of all breast cancers. Another study published in the American Journal of Epidemiology found that women have a 20% reduced chance of getting cancer if they follow a similar healthy diet.

A poor diet is one filled with lots of fats, especially unhealthy refined oils, refined maida-based products such as patties, pastries, biscuits, and bread. Some junk and processed foods have been so highly refined that they have been totally stripped of any nutrients and are laden with additives and chemicals, some known to be carcinogens. In addition, processed foods are often wrapped in plastic, which contains cancer-causing BPA.

How does food affect our immune system?

To better understand why and how we should be eating better to combat cancer and other diseases, it is important to understand the meanings of the terms immune system, inflammation, oxidative stress, and free radicals, which are all factors that play key roles in the development and growth of cancer.

The human body has been gifted with an immune system that gives the body the ability to ward off disease. The immune system comprises of cells and organs that work together to protect the body and respond to infection and disease. When the immune system is triggered to defend the body against infection and disease, it is called the immune response. One of the major causes of cellular injury and death is damage from **free radicals** or **oxidative stress**. Free radicals are associated with many human diseases, including cancer, atherosclerosis, Alzheimer's disease, and Parkinson's disease. There is also a link between free radicals and aging, a process defined as a "gradual accumulation of free-radical damage."

Free radicals are the natural byproducts of the body's metabolic processes and are formed in everyone's body. In small amounts, free radicals are beneficial. It is only when there is an excessive amount generated that they become

Avoid refined flour to reduce Cancer risk
Most bakery products such as bread, biscuits, toasts, pastries as well as roomali rotis, some tandoori rotis are mostly made from white refined flour (maida). Studies have found that this flour is devoid of many nutrients. For example, it lacks the minimum amount of selenium which reduces the risk of prostate cancer. Selenium is abundant in whole grains and pulses.

Substances that produce free radicals can be found in the food we eat, the medicines we take, the air we breathe, and the water we drink. These include tobacco smoke, alcohol, fried foods, and pesticides.

dangerous and lead to cellular injury. Free radicals are simply single electrons searching for a partner to pair with. These single "bachelor" electrons move around the body in large numbers causing disharmony and damage. This can lead to premature aging of the skin, eyes, liver, heart, lungs, brain, and more. Excessive free radicals in the body give rise to inflammation of the blood vessels, joints, and intestines.

Those more prone to free radical damage are people who:

- Smoke
- Drink excessively
- Live in polluted cities
- Have constant exposure to infections
- Are under chronic stress
- Have a heavy intake of junk food
- Have a diet deficient in vitamins and minerals
- Perform excessive physical activity (laborers, athletes)

So how does inflammation lead to cancer?

The Latin root of the word inflammation is *"inflammare,"* which means "to set on fire." Inflammation is a normal physiological response that helps cells and tissues heal. The process works like this: chemicals are released by damaged tissues that cause white blood cells to make substances that cause cells to divide and grow to rebuild tissue as a way to help repair the injury. Swelling around an injury on your ankle, for example, is an inflammatory response. Once the ankle is healed, the inflammatory process ends.

When inflammation is chronic, the inflammatory process occurs even if there is no injury, and so it serves no healing purpose. This happens mostly internally and is often caused by oxidative stress. It is not always known why the inflammation continues, but various conditions can cause oxidative stress. These include persistent infections, cell growth due to obesity, or abnormal reactions to normal tissues. **Over time, this chronic inflammation can cause DNA damage and lead to cancer.** For example, those with chronic inflammatory pancreatitis have an increased risk of pancreatic cancer.

Ultra-processed food increased risk of overall Cancers by 12%
Findings published in the British medical journal Clinical Nutrition based on an extensive survey found that ultraprocessed foods like pizza, chicken nuggets, cake, biscuits, chips, and other savoury packaged snacks increased the risk of overall cancer by 12%. Carcinogenic contaminants and additives like sodium nitrite, titanium oxide etc. have been found in processed food products which have been made using high heat (i.e., majority of processed foods) (Isaksen & Dankel, 2023).

How can I control my free radical damage?

The best natural tools to control free radical damage are antioxidants present in certain foods. Antioxidants are exactly what the words mean: working against oxidants or oxidation primarily caused by free radicals. These molecules bind to these free radicals preventing their ability to damage cells, potentially improving health. Our diet should include plenty of antioxidants.

> *Say no to processed meat*
> *A study of 190,000 people found that those who eat large quantities of processed minced meat like sausages and hot dogs had the highest rate of pancreatic cancer. Lower your risk by buying and preparing unprocessed meats and prepare them using traditional cooking methods.*

Four major vitamins and minerals are classified as antioxidants: vitamin C, vitamin E, selenium, and beta-carotene, which are converted to vitamin A in the body. In addition to these main nutrients, many phytonutrients or plant nutrients also act as antioxidants. These include flavonoids and polyphenols. The phytonutrients within all these categories are numerous. There are more than 600 known carotenoids alone. Each food source for antioxidants has a unique set of these phytonutrients, and nutrition research regularly discovers new compounds and health benefits. The downside to this is the hype created around antioxidants. Any compound with antioxidant action is instantly put in a pill form and marketed to the public as the healthy pill you cannot live without.

In fact, getting antioxidants from food is preferred over loading up on supplements. Research on the effectiveness of these supplements is mixed, and it is possible to get too much of these vitamins and minerals, which can lead to toxicity. Having a variety of foods on your *thali* ensures a healthy balance of antioxidants. **Plant-based food like fruits and vegetables, along with nuts, legumes, and whole grains, are the best sources of antioxidants.**

Foods with high ORAC scores are especially high in antioxidants. ORAC stands for Oxygen Radical Absorbance Capacity, which is a lab technique used to quantify the total antioxidant capacity of a food. The test is performed by placing a food sample (for example, cinnamon), in a test tube combined with certain molecules that generate free radical activity. After some time, the scientist measures how well cinnamon protects the susceptible molecules from oxidation. The less free radical damage there is, the higher the antioxidant capacity of the food and, therefore, the higher the ORAC score.

Indian Foods with high ORAC value

Food	ORAC Value
Triphala powder	706250
Dried gooseberries(*amla*)	261500
Sorghum (*jowar*)	24000
Cinnamon (*dalchini*)	131420
Nutmeg (*jaiphal*)	69640
Dried basil (*sabja*)	61063
Cumin seeds (*jeera*)	50372
Ground ginger (*saunth*)	39041
Chavanpravash	35700
Black pepper	34053
Chili powder	23636
Golden raisins	10450
Ashwagandha root, dried	8487
Turmeric (*haldi*)	159277
Moringa (drumstick)	157600
Cloves, ground	314446

Cancer Prevention through the Indian Thali

What is a *Thali?*

The Indian *thali* is an Instagram-worthy sight: an assortment of shiny steel *katoris* (small steel bowls) filled with varied foods adorning a large round platter. The word *thali* came from the Hindi word *thal,* which simply means plate. For centuries, basic everyday food in India has been a balanced mixture of grains, vegetables, dals, and pulses, adapted to regional preferences. For example, *rotis* (bread) is made with the local staple: wheat, *jowar* (sorghum), *bajra* (pearl millet) in the North, and rice and *ragi* (finger millet) in the South. Vegetables were local, and very little was shipped in. No plates or cutlery were required – food was eaten with one's hands and served on banana or *pathravali* leaves (from the sal tree) before steel plates became popular.

The use of *katoris* followed the plates made with leaves. The word *donas* or small bowls can be found in texts from the Vedic period. The portions in a *thali* depended upon the composition of the food and the economic condition of the community. There is a standard method of serving food on the *thali*: salt, pickle, chutneys, and *papadam* (thin cracker, roasted or fried) are always served first in order on the left side of the plate. These items are to ignite the digestive fire and promote the appetite. They are generally not needed to be served as seconds.

The vegetables, pulses, and curries, all made using healing spices such as turmeric, cumin, and cinnamon, are served next in the individual *katoris*. Rotis, rice, and some dal to top the rice are served next. Tradition dictates that staples – rice or roti – depending on the part of the country, are never served on an empty plate, and condiments and vegetables are always served first.

To most Indian people today, the word *thali* conjures the thought of the restaurant thali with numerous items on the plate and several bowls holding various foods. But these *thalis* are far different than traditional ones. Restaurant *thalis* can be unhealthy because the foods that are usually made in large quantities often use cheaper oils for faster cooking. There are always fried items and sweets included on these thalis, which is not something you should have very often. Like all restaurant foods, more fat is added to dishes to make them tastier.

Research shows that the greater the variety of foods, the more you will eat. That's why we overeat at a buffet. If a thali has 10 items and you have a few bites of each, you will have had quite a bit. Often times the restaurant thali is unlimited, just like a buffet – the server keeps coming around to see if you want more of any item and you take seconds or thirds of the dishes you like. There is absolutely no portion control.

Additionally, numerous *katoris* filled with a variety of *sabjis* (vegetables), dals, and curries rest on the plate in restaurant *thalis*, an assortment you would not have at home. Who can cook so many dishes for everyday meals?

The traditional *thali* eaten every day in our homes is not nearly as elaborate as the restaurant *thali*, but offers balanced nutrition with the right mix of macronutrients (carbs, protein, and fat) and micronutrients (vitamins and minerals). Rotis or rice are the staple grains, dals, pulses, and curds are the protein sources, and vegetables offer vitamins, minerals, and fiber. Fermented foods like *dahi* (yoghurt) and *chaas* (buttermilk) give the probiotic or good gut bacteria advantage, and *dahi* also is an excellent source of calcium and protein. Fermented foods also help increase the absorption of needed vitamins from the gastrointestinal tract, thus preventing vitamin deficiencies. This is not to be confused with pickles, which are not usually fermented, as is the common belief. Pickling began at a time when there was no refrigeration and a need to preserve seasonal vegetables. Most pickles are preserved, not fermented, so they do not contain any enzymes to help with the gut. Most Indian pickles use salt and oil for preservation. Even though you need to cure pickles for 10-15 days, no fermentation occurs, and the added salt and oil do not allow for fermentation. Pickles do play a role, however; they stimulate the appetite. Our mothers gave us pickles with curd rice when we were ill so we would gain some appetite.

The food you begin and end your meal with on the *thali* depends on the part of the country you are in. In Gujarat and Maharashtra, a small *katori* of a sweet dish comes as the first course. *Chaas* or buttermilk comes last. In Karnataka, curd rice is served at the end of the meal after the dessert of *payasam*. In Bengal, *shukto*, a spicy dish made with bitter gourd starts the meal. They believe that a bitter taste enhances the appetite. These practices are seldom seen in homes these days, but they come alive during weddings and festivals. However, there are many common denominators of the *thali* across the country, such as:

- The use of seasonal and local ingredients
- A balance of nutrients
- The liberal use of healing spices

- A balance of portions
- Traditional ways of cooking slowly on a low flame
- The use of tempering (tadka)

Tadka

In colloquial Hindi, the term *tadka* is used to imply someone adding spice to a conversation. *Tadka* is just that – added spice. *Tadkas* are the basis of Indian cuisine, usually added at the beginning of the cooking process but it can also be sprinkled as a finishing touch on top of the dish, which is more common in South Indian dishes.

Tadka is a process in which ghee or oil is heated to a certain temperature and various herbs and spices are added to it. Dals, curries, sabjis and various rice preparations in Indian cuisine all use *tadkas*.

A typical *tadka* is created in 3 steps:

1. Oil or pure ghee is heated
2. Various herbs and spices are added one after another. These may include cumin seeds, mustard seeds, curry leaves, garlic, red/green chilies, turmeric, asafetida. In some preparations, spices like cloves, pepper, cinnamon, cardamom, and bay leaf are also added. The inclusion or exclusion of the *tadka* ingredients depends on the spice meter of the dish.
3. Once the spices pop and sizzle, other ingredients are added. Sometimes the *tadka* is put on a prepared dish as a finishing touch. Please note that for tempering, the oil or ghee needs to be cooked at high temperature. Therefore, oil with a low smoke point such as olive oil cannot be used.

This tempering of spices and herbs is not just for taste and flavor. Nutritionists believe that there are many health benefits of the *tadka* technique, including the fact that *tadka* unlocks the full flavor potential of spices, thus making the dish more aromatic.

In the case of some ailments, including cancer, patients develop dyspepsia (loss of appetite), resulting in physical weakness due to lack of food. A fine *tadka* not only makes the dish more appealing to the senses but also increases one's appetite and helps combat dyspepsia with the action of the spices.

- When *tadka* is added to the dish, the oil helps the body absorb fat soluble vitamins (A, D, E, and K) from the food.
- It is believed that the process of *tadka* unlocks the healing properties of the spices and herbs. The essential oils and beneficial components present in the spices are released in the heated oil.
- A study showed that when spices like turmeric and pepper were cooked for 30 minutes the curcumin in turmeric and capsaicin in pepper were lost to the tune of 60-90%. But when the spices were tempered, the active medicinal ingredients were retained (Bhide, 2011).

The dishes in the *thali* offer an assortment of textures and flavors to satisfy the senses. When you read further in this book, you will see that the *thali* has all the elements needed for an anti-cancer diet, including probiotics, prebiotics, fiber, and plenty of phytochemicals from vegetables, dals, and spices.

The Science of the Indian *Thali*

It has long been known that plant-based diets have vast nutritional benefits. Recent nutrition research on phytochemicals found in plant foods uncovered exactly how these compounds are beneficial. These include abundant phytochemicals that promote healthy and diverse gut microbiota, reduce intestinal and systemic inflammation, and decrease the risk of colorectal cancer and type 2 diabetes mellitus.

Fibers found in whole grains and various *sabjis* of the *thali* are crucial to a healthy diet. Fiber binds itself to estrogen, preventing it from feeding tumor cells and making it very effective in preventing cancer. Archaeological evidence of grain agriculture, including several wheat and barley varieties, has been found in excavations dated to the sixth millennium BC (Kajale, 1974). Development of this grain cultivation early in the ancient Indus Valley has allowed India to experiment with food and find crops suitable to its needs.

The importance of prebiotics should be stressed as well. Prebiotics lay the groundwork for probiotics to work and are the non-digestible fiber part of foods, mostly found in vegetables and pulses. Prebiotic fiber goes through the small intestine undigested and is fermented when it reaches the large intestine. This fermentation process feeds beneficial bacteria colonies (including probiotic bacteria) and helps to increase the number of beneficial bacteria in our gut that lead to better health and reduced risk. Although all the items on the *thali* play a role in cancer protection, prebiotics is the main item that makes it cancer protective. On the other hand, the Western diet generally includes very few vegetables, creating a less healthy environment for the digestive system. Prebiotic elements make the *thali* unique and nourishing, promoting an anti-disease environment in the body.

Our *thali* is a combination of many tastes and colors. Each pigment, green, yellow, purple, red, orange, and yellow, has certain valuable bioactive compounds beneficial to health. The thali ideally should be filled with this colorful rainbow and tweaked every day to get the goodness of the variety of plant foods available.

Here are examples of this plant-based rainbow diet:

Red   : *Beets, Rajgira leaves (lal math), Chili peppers, Red Capsicum, Pomegranate, Radish, Red Apple, Strawberries, Tomatoes, Watermelon*

Red fruits and veggies have vitamin A (beta carotene), vitamin C, manganese, and fiber. Apples have quercetin, a compound helpful in avoiding cancer. Capsicum and chili peppers have powerful anti-inflammatory agents. Lycopene present in tomatoes is an anti-cancer compound.

Orange : *Carrots, Musk Melon, Papaya, Mango, Apricot, Orange, Sweet Lime, Peach, Pumpkin, and Sweet Potatoes*

The Alpha and beta-carotenes present in plants are potent anti-cancer agents. Beta-carotenes play a role in reducing lung, esophagus, and stomach cancer risks.

Yellow : *Corn, Lemon, Yellow capsicum, Pears, Pineapple, and Banana*

Orange and yellow fruits and veggies have antioxidant vitamin C. Citrus fruits, particularly carrots, contain vitamin A (beta-carotene) for improved eyesight. They also contain potassium, fiber, and vitamin B6 for general health support. Yellow fruits and veggies have manganese, potassium, vitamin A, fiber, and magnesium. Turmeric, the well-known spice of India, is found to have a strong resistance against the growth of cancer cells.

Purple : *Brinjal, Fig, Jamun, Purple grapes, Purple plums, and Purple sweet potatoes*

Purple fruits and veggies have anthocyanins and resveratrol, powerful antioxidants that protect the blood vessels from breakage and prevent the destruction of collagen, a protein, for healthy skin. Nutrients in these vegetables are rich in vitamin A and flavonoids.

Black : *Indian blackberries like karvand and tutti, Dates, Mushrooms, Black currents, Black grapes, Black olives, Black plums*

Black fruits and veggies have a variety of nutrients, including B vitamins, selenium, potassium, and copper. Mushrooms also have vitamin D.

Green : *Cabbage, Capsicum, Celery, Coriander, Cucumbers, Green apples, French beans, Green grapes, Green pears, Green* *tomatoes, Green melon, Leafy greens, Lettuce, Okra, Peas, Spinach, Spring onions, other leafy greens, and assorted green herbs*

Green veggies, especially dark green leafy ones, act as antioxidants in the body. An excellent source of fiber, folate, and carotenoids, these vegetables also contain vitamins C and K and iron and calcium minerals. Cruciferous vegetables like cabbage are rich in isothiocyanates and indole, phytochemicals that have anti-cancer properties.

Green vegetables that are not typically in the *thali* meal but can be included in other meals are Arugula, Asparagus, Avocados, Bok choy, Broccoli, Zucchini, and Green olives.

Other Beneficial Nutrients in the Thali

1. Omega-3s

Omega-3s are a type of polyunsaturated fatty acid (PuFA) found to be heart and brain protective. Our body does not produce omega-3 on its own, hence the need to provide them through diet or supplements. Omega-3s also protect joints from degeneration, regulate mood, protect from depression, and help balance hormones. Researchers believe that due to the potent anti-inflammatory properties of Omega-3s, they can offer protection from many types of cancers.

Vegetable Sources (ALA)	Animal Sources (DHA, EPA, ETA)
Green Leafy Vegetables	Egg Yolk
Flax seeds	Fish like cod, sardines, tuna, salmon, mackerel
Chia Seeds	
Walnuts	
Soybean or Canola oil (not recommended)	

2. Probiotics

Gut health is basically the premise of Ayurveda, India's 5,000-year-old science, and today's health sector seems to be catching on. Probiotics, a beneficial form of gut bacteria, are currently a buzzword in healthy eating circles, and with good reason, as they have been found to offer protection from certain cancers and are touted as the key to gastrointestinal stability, brain health, and even heart health.

The Indian diet contains many probiotic foods. *Dahi* and buttermilk are universal, and foods made from fermented batters like *dosas, idlis, dhokla, and kanji vadas* (depending on which part of India you are from) are all part of our daily diet. The importance of digestion and gut health can be seen on the *thali* as several probiotic foods – *Dahi* (yogurt), *chaas* (buttermilk), and *raita* (salad with yogurt) are integral components.

Beneficial gut bacteria also protect us from auto-immune diseases and help keep our digestive system and immunity in excellent condition by preventing harmful bacteria from colonizing. Research has found that a high amount of beneficial gut bacteria keeps us calm and helps activate the rational part of the brain more than the emotional part (Lee *et al*, 2020). Studies show that more than 70% of our serotonin (happy hormone) is made in our gut with the help of beneficial gut bacteria (*ibid.*). Probiotics help offset medications, bad food choices, stress, and aging, which can deplete the good bacteria in the gut. Other damaging factors are X-rays and other medical procedures, such as radiation during treatment. Taking probiotics also helps with the side effects of chemotherapy, especially diarrhea.

Prebiotics are types of dietary fiber that feed the friendly bacteria in the gut. Prebiotic foods are also needed to enhance the action of probiotic foods. These include whole grains, bananas, garlic, onions, cabbage, radish, potatoes, and cauliflower; basically high fiber, plant-based foods.

One randomized trial found that patients who underwent chemotherapy and received probiotics experienced significantly less grade three and four diarrhea and required fewer hospitalizations and dose reductions due to bowel toxicity (Wei *et al*, 2018).

According to Stacy Kennedy, MPH, RD, a senior clinical nutritionist at Dana-Farber/Brigham and Women's Cancer Center, probiotics can also be beneficial for patients with preexisting health problems such as irritable bowel syndrome, as well as those experiencing other gastrointestinal issues like constipation, gas, or bloating. Kennedy also recommends that these patients vary the types of probiotics they consume to benefit from a variety of probiotic strains.

Evidence shows that fermented foods are also excellent for helping with long term symptom management for cancer patients following treatment, especially those related to diarrhea. Several studies have shown a decrease in symptoms for patients suffering from colorectal cancer as well. You should include traditional probiotic foods in your daily diet (Eslami et al, 2019).

However, probiotics are not the holy grail of natural meds for healthy gut maintenance or improving gastrointestinal problems. Fibers from fruits and vegetables, nuts, and whole-grain foods are also needed to maintain and improve overall gut health. Vegetables are still the most important part of the *thali*.

Probiotic foods are natural immune boosters, and we are fortunate to have many of them included as part of our *thali*. Please note that not all packaged *dahi* from grocery stores contain probiotics. Commercialized

> *Some gastrointestinal issues that patients may experience, such as gas, can also be caused from beverages like carbonated soda, which can create a buildup of gas in the abdominal area. You may think you are healing your gut by drinking soda, but in fact, it may be detrimental.*

dahis use high-temperature treatment to kill off any harmful bacteria in the milk, a process that can also cause good bacteria to disappear. Probiotic cultures are very sensitive to heat and will not survive pasteurization. Even making *dahi* at home is a high-level skill as creating a really good, creamy *dahi* requires the right milk temperature adjusted to the temperature of the atmosphere and adding just the right amount of live culture.

If you have an abnormal blood cell count, you should ask your doctor before taking any probiotic supplementation.

3. Chutneys

Chutneys are super-healthy Indian add-ons that have existed in our culture for centuries. We have yet to come across a chutney recipe that is harmful to health. There are numerous types, ranging from radish, carrot, wood apple, green tomato, and red tomatoes; the list is quite long. Chutneys need very little preparation time — just get the ingredients together and grind. Dry chutneys have a good shelf life, stimulate taste buds, and are excellent for packaged lunches. They were once must-haves on the Indian *thali*, but taste buds have changed through the years and these nutritious power bombs have been replaced by sugary or salty alternatives like jam, sauces, ketchup, mayonnaise, and sandwich spreads — all highly processed and full of unhealthy chemicals and preservatives.

The Anti-Cancer Indian *thali* cannot be complete without a spoonful of dry or wet chutney. Consider it your daily dietary supplement. Here are a few examples of chutneys and their nutritional benefits.

Chutney	Benefits
Groundnut (Peanut) Garlic Chutney	High protein, increases level of good cholesterol
Flaxseed Chutney	Natural supply of omega-3s, heart protective, good for joints, beneficial for menopausal women
Sesame Chutney	High protein, high calcium, heart protective
Curry Leaves Chutney	High calcium, rich in antioxidants, helps in anorexia
Garlic Chutney	Heart protective, reduces cholesterol, cancer protective
Coconut Chutney	Beneficial for weakness, fatigue, and natural weight gain
Mint Chutney	Beneficial in anorexia, nausea, dyspepsia
Tamarind Chutney	Helps in combating dyspepsia and metallic taste
Ridge gourd Chutney	Made with the peels; Very high fiber, antioxidant rich
Coriander Chutney	Coriander leaves and lemon have alkaline properties. Chilies and garlic are cancer protective

4. Protein

Protein on a balanced vegetarian thali will be sufficient if you consciously include your dals, pulses, and *dahi*. An average 60kg adult who is moderately active needs about 48 grams of protein (.8g of protein x 60kg). One *katori* of dal (12g) + one *katori* pulses (12g) + one *katori* dahi (8g) = 32 grams of protein. Each *katori* is 150ml of volume, slightly more than half a cup. This does not include the protein in other ingredients such as wheat, jowar, groundnuts, cashews, and sesame seeds which are often used in cooking.

During cancer treatment and recovery, protein intake may need to increase. Protein is needed for cell repair and growth and is important to maintain a healthy immune system.

Vegetarians may need protein supplementation. Include proteins in your snack foods as well with these high-protein snacks such as Dahi, Lassi, Roasted chana dal, Muthiya (savory snack), Sprout salad, Cheela (savory pancake), Chana chaat, Pumpkin Seeds, Nuts (almonds and pistachios), Peanuts, Hard-boiled eggs, Nut butter (peanut) with fruit/veggies, Protein shake, Baked tofu, Roasted paneer, Hummus and veggies, 2 cubes of unprocessed cheese with fruit, Kothimbir Vadi, Dhokla, Appe with Chutney, Idli with Chutney.

What to Include in your Thali?

Ensure you have this on your *thali*:

- 50% of the *thali* should be vegetables, cooked and raw.
- 25% should be proteins: pulses, dal, legumes, paneer, or non-veg in the form of free-range chicken, fish, eggs, or mutton.
- 20% should be whole grains and millets.
- 5% or less should be Indian traditional probiotics and Indian oil seed chutneys.

Why do we need to provide specific proportions for the *thalis* we have been eating for centuries? There are two reasons. First, our homemade *thalis* have changed through the years. Dairy, non-veg, and sweets once laced the plate only on special occasions, but now have become more affordable and are often many times more prominent on the plate than healthy vegetables. Secondly, the roti/rice to vegetable proportion can no longer remain the same as it was for our grandparents. With our sedentary lifestyles, we simply do not burn as many calories as they did. Walking, gymming, or working out for an hour a few times a week does not constitute enough calorie expenditure for the amount of carbs that continue to dominate the *thali*.

The proportions offered by us provide an important dietary tool for cancer prevention. All the foods on a thali made in our traditional Indian way form a cancer-protective environment in the body that continues to work after treatment as well. This *thali* can also protect one from other diseases such as:

- Type 2 diabetes
- Hypertension
- Obesity
- Other lifestyle diseases like dyslipidemia, hypothyroidism, etc.

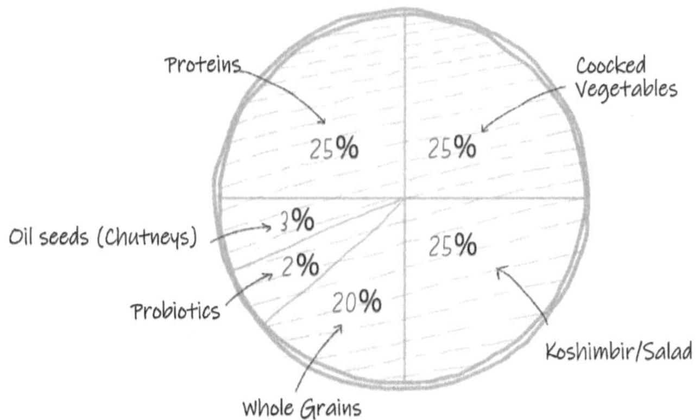

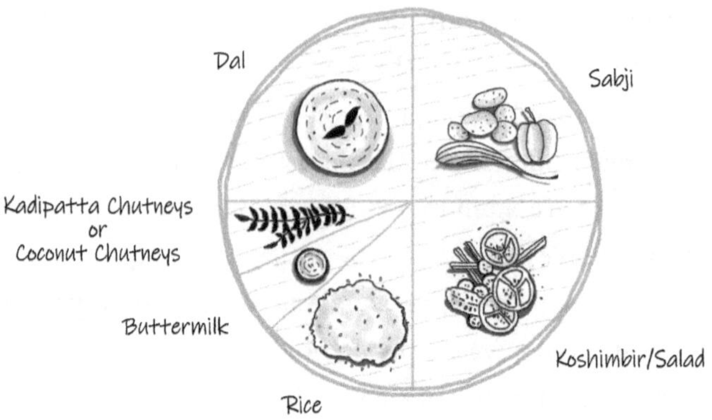
Dal
Sabji
Kadipatta Chutneys
or
Coconut Chutneys
Buttermilk
Koshimbir/Salad
Rice

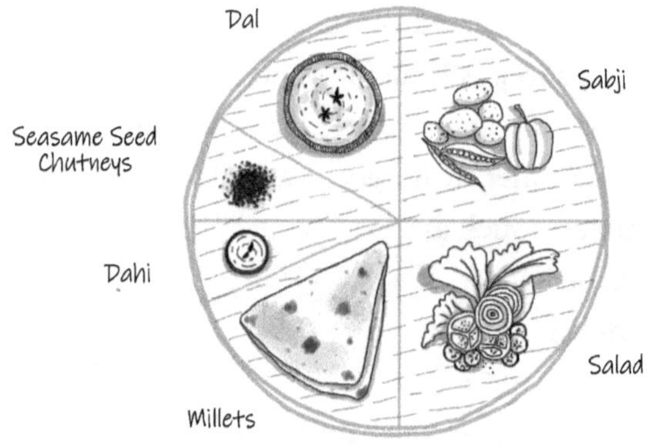
Dal
Sabji
Seasame Seed
Chutneys
Dahi
Salad
Millets

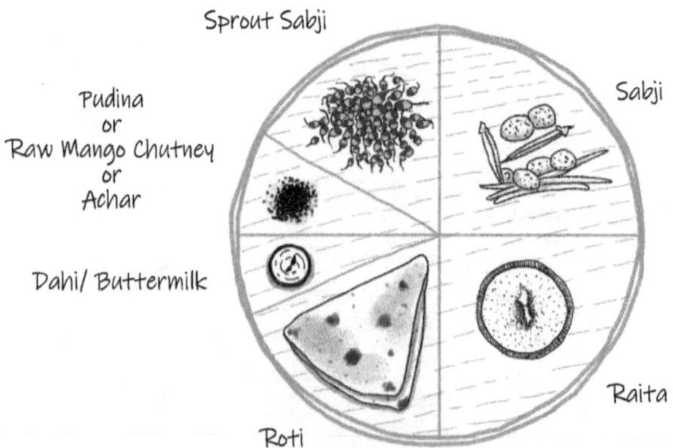
Sprout Sabji
Pudina
or
Raw Mango Chutney
or
Achar
Sabji
Dahi/ Buttermilk
Raita
Roti

The Mediterranean diet, which is considered the healthiest diet in the world today, has similar proportions as the *thali* we've recommended.

In the earlier chapters, we have urged following the 80-20% rule when it comes to your diet. Eat well 80% of the time, and other 20%, you are allowed to indulge in foods that are not so healthy. That means that 8 out of 10 meals should be healthy. And remember eating healthy is in no way a punishment. Your body will start feeling lighter and more energetic, and you won't feel like eating junk food. You'll begin to appreciate the taste of real food and relish the dishes on the thali.

Your nutritional goals can be met if you adhere to the following principles:

- Avoid simple carbohydrates – basically, any *maida*-based foods. Instead, eat and cook with whole grains such as whole wheat, bajra, jowar, ragi, rice, and rajgeera.
- Avoid processed foods – foods that come in packages contain chemicals and preservatives, even those that claim they are "made with grains" or "all natural".
- Limit sugar.
- Avoid junk or fast food. Chain stores sell burgers, pizza, chicken, and other kinds of food made with loads of fats, low-quality meats, and *maida*.
- Cook more and eat more homemade foods.
- Avoid trans fats, saturated fats, and too much animal fat.
- Avoid red meat and processed meat.
- Avoid alcohol.
- Increase your intake of vegetables, pulses, and dals.
- Increase fiber.
- Use herbs and spices in cooking.

A homemade *thali* incorporates all of the above. We explore this in the coming chapter.

♦♦♦

Thoughts on Junk

"These trans fatty acids Walk through your body like Frankenstein, terrorizing your metabolism."

– Robert Crayhon,
Nutrition for Longer Life

"Eating Sugar is like hitting yourself in head with a baseball bat. The less you do it, the better."

– Robert Crayhon,
Nutrition for Longer Life

"Fast food is about as destructive and evil as it gets. It celebrates the mentality of sloth, convenience and cheerful embrace of food we know is hurting us."

– Anthony Bourdain,
Chef

"Get people back into kitchen and combat the trend. toward processed food & fast food."

– Andrew Weil,
MD

"As a chef and father, it kills me that children are fed processed foods, foods loaded with preservatives and high fructose com syrup."

– Jose Andres,
Chef

Gems of the Indian Kitchen

"Superfoods" is a term you read often in the context of wonder foods that are the elixir of health. But, there are no real super foods, and there are no foods you eat in isolation that can ward off cancer. Health companies and big pharma try and market the next healthiest nutrient into a concentrated pill form but pills are not the best way to get the benefits of these foods. The human body absorbs nutrients in minute doses and these doses interact with other ingredients that you take. A well-balanced diet that includes a variety of foods with high ORAC values, and that have anti-inflammatory effects is the healthiest option. You don't have to look too far – many can be found on the *thali*. There are an abundance of fruits and vegetables available in India, all helping with creating an optimally healthy environment in the body. We have chosen the following top ten as "Indian Gems." They have been chosen because they are all indigenous to India, available all over India, and fairly affordable. Other than *haldi* (turmeric) all the items on the list have a whole spectrum of various nutrients, thus giving a good package of health. And finally, they are comfort foods – we as Indians have grown up with these foods and have a psychological attachment to these ingredients and foods made with them.

Turmeric (Haldi)

Turmeric, which has been a part of the Indian diet for centuries is now touted world over as the wonder spice. Here in India, we have always used *haldi* for medicinal purposes – warm haldi doodh (turmeric milk) is the first thing a mother gives her child when they have to soothe a sore throat. A paste of *haldi* is applied to help a wound to heal and the same paste is applied to brighten the skin of the bride in a *haldi* ceremony the day before the wedding.

The medical and scientific community as well as culinary enthusiasts have recently discovered turmeric's antioxidant and anti-inflammatory effects. They are specifically interested in curcumin, the active bio-compound that has medicinal properties. Research specific to curcumin's role in metabolic syndromes, arthritis, anxiety, dementia and the reduction of exercise-induced inflammation and muscle soreness and much more are ongoing. There are hundreds of studies being conducted on curcumin's role in suppressing tumors and cell growth.

The medical community is concerned about poor bioavailability of curcumin, which means we cannot absorb in our bodies as much as we would like. Piperine is the major active component of black pepper and, when combined with curcumin, has been shown to increase bioavailability by 2000% (Shoba *et al*, 1997). Hence, turmeric supplements usually include piperine as well. In Indian cooking, black pepper and *haldi* are the ingredients (along with many other healthy spices) in most curry powders or masalas, both homemade and commercial. Our bodies have been slowly ingesting these active compounds over years and reaping the benefits. At least one or two dishes on the *thali* will have *haldi*.

Amla

Amla, the Indian Gooseberry, is mentioned in ancient Ayurvedic texts with great reverence. It is called 'dhatri phal' which means, 'caretaker for life'. Amla is the only food that has 5 of the 6 Ayurvedic tastes (sweet, salty, sour, bitter, pungent, astringent) with only salty being missing. This rare quality of amla promotes longevity. Although all berries are considered cancer protective, amla has been studied with larger interest due to its high tannin content and antioxidant properties. It also has the highest ORAC value in the fruit category. Both invitro and in vivo studies done on this fruit strongly refer to its potent anti-cancer properties. These properties have been attributed to the high content of flavonoids and tannins like ellagic acid and gallic acid, amongst others. Amla has a high amount of Vitamin C – more than any other fruit. Gallic acid present in amla protects the vitamin C in this fruit, which means drying, cooking, or storing amla does not decrease its vitamin C content, it is bio-protected. Amla powder is available all over India at a very economical price and it too has a high amount of Vitamin C. Alkaline in nature, there is substantial scientific evidence that amla has strong anti-inflammatory properties, supporting its anti-cancer activity.

Amla fruit is available in the Indian Market during October till February. It can be directly eaten with a sprinkle of salt or can be grated fresh and added to salads, kohshimbiris and raitas. Dried amla powder can be taken one teaspoon a day with warm water or honey.

Tulsi (Holy Basil)

A *tulsi* plant adorns the garden of every home in specially designed pots. Holy basil or *tulsi* is sacred and holds religious significance in India. It is commonly used in pujas (Hindu rituals) and infused in tea to help with colds and coughs. *Tulsi* is anti-inflammatory, loaded with antioxidants and therefore cancer protective. With its anti-bacterial, anti-fungal, anti-depressive and skin rejuvenation qualities, it has been a favorite of naturopaths and Ayurvedic practitioners for generations. With its anti-inflammatory properties it has attracted the attention of cancer researchers as well. Studies in animals has shown that the holy basil seed oil can slow down progression of many types of cancers. The antioxidant ability of the oil is seen to benefit the survival rate in certain types of cancers in animals. These properties also help healthy cells from toxicity during radiation and chemotherapy.

Nutritionally, *tulsi* has calcium, copper, iron, magnesium, potassium, phosphorus, sodium, vitamin K and zinc. It has potent antioxidants like selenium, vitamin C and beta carotene. *Tulsi* oil has phytochemicals in the form of eugenol, ursolic acid, oleanolic acid and many more. Use it in salads, soups, raitas and any dish where you would like the flavor. You can also flavor your water with *tulsi* for a few hours to make a refreshing drink.

Garlic

The American Institute for Cancer Research (AICR) is a reputed body conducting and compiling cancer research. The AICR has found that eating garlic regularly lowers the risk of colorectal cancers. Compounds found in garlic help to

> ### *Cooked & Uncooked Garlic*
>
> *The potent anticancer properties of garlic can be made available in two ways: either eating raw, peeled garlic cloves daily or by adding garlic cloves to all your meal preparations (sabzi, dal etc.). Before chopping up vegetables and kneading flour, the first task you should do is peel garlic cloves and let them sit on the kitchen top for about 15 minutes. Alliinase, an enzyme in garlic, which has strong anticancer properties takes some time to develop the chemical reaction. If you peel and immediately throw the cloves in heated oil, the alliinase gets inactivated thus stopping the cancer protective chemical reaction.*

slow the growth of cancer cells, decrease inflammation and help with DNA repair. Each clove is packed with numerous phytochemicals, many of which have cancer fighting properties (allicin). While the research that garlic lowers colorectal risk is the strongest, garlic is also being studied for its role in reducing risk for other cancers as well.

Ginger

Ginger is a staple in every Indian home, both for cooking and to address gastrointestinal issues. In addition to easing an upset stomach, the juice of ginger mixed with honey works wonders for a congested chest. *Adrak ki chai* (ginger tea) is commonly had during the rains to ward off the cold. Ginger is in fact listed 13th on the most impressive antioxidant list with an ORAC score of 28,811 (see Chapter 2 for more information about ORAC values). It has been found to inhibit tumor cell growth, suppress metastasis, provide protection from carcinogenic agents in the liver, support a natural immune response, inhibit inflammation, and enhance chemotherapeutic drugs.

Drumstick (Moringa)

Every part of the drumstick plant is beneficial for health, from the leaves and the flowers of the tree as well as the meaty vegetable itself. Today moringa, particularly the leaves of the plant, are a health rage – moringa leaf powder is added to tea, smoothies, soups and oatmeal. While the world celebrates moringa leaves and moringa powder as superfoods, take note that the stalks and flowers are equally powerful, and have always been part of the *thali*. *Sabjis* and cutlets are foods made with moringa leaves and flowers in addition to the actual drumstick itself.

Drumsticks contain a variety of vital nutrients. They are rich in B vitamins like thiamine, riboflavin and niacin, all good for the skin and hair. The folic acid is also good for pregnant women. Drumsticks also offer the benefits of vitamin A, like eye health and skin rejuvenation. For bone health, drumsticks are rich in two vital nutrients – calcium and iron. Drumsticks also have digestive properties, helping the liver, and stomach issues like constipation, colitis and acidity, all making it colon cancer protective.

Gourd Family Vegetables

The Gourd Family of vegetables include ash gourd (*kohla*), bitter gourd (*karela*), ridge gourd (*dodka*), snake gourd (*padwal/chachinda*), smooth gourd (*ghosale/torai*), bottle gourd (*lauki*), red pumpkin (*kaddu*) and *parwar* along with a host of regional varieties.

All gourds are climber plants and predominantly alkaline. Every region in India has its own way of preparing *sabjis* from these vegetables. They can also be added to parathas, pancakes, and raitas (yogurt-based salads). Gourds are high in iron, copper and essential minerals. Their antioxidants and several anti-inflammatory compounds coupled with their alkaline nature make gourds anti-cancer. Research published in 2016 has found a novel anti-cancer peptide in bitter gourd which showed cytotoxic effect in colon cancer cells in humans (Dia & Krishnan, 2016). Researchers have also found that crude extract of bitter gourd inhibits proliferation of breast, prostate and pancreatic cancer cells. Gourds are rich in insoluble and soluble dietary fiber, which researchers believe help create an anti-cancer environment in the body due their pre-biotic activity (Sharma *et al*, 2021). In our private practices we have observed that while undergoing cancer treatment, patients are able to tolerate the gourd family *sabjis* easily. Gourds did not create any unfavorable symptoms like acidity, diarrhea, or constipation which can occur during chemo and radiation. We recommend eating a variety of gourds during treatment and also for cancer prevention.

Makhana (Fox Nut)

This wonder snack is popular in North India. In fact, 80% of makhana is cultivated in Bihar. These seeds go through a series of natural processes (drying, roasting, polishing) before it is packed and distributed. The traditional method of preparing *makhana* from seeds does not involve any use of chemicals so plain, non-flavored makhana, can be considered a nutritious, alkaline, easily digestible, precooked snack full of antioxidants. *Makhana* is a good source of omega -3 fatty acids and good minerals such as copper, magnesium, and phosphorus. *Makhana* is beneficial during cancer therapy as it is quite digestible, does not have a strong flavor and does not need prep time.

Coconut

Every part of the coconut is useful. This is why coconuts are termed 'shrifal', the fruit of prosperity, and used in religious ceremonies. Even after the water, milk, and flesh are used, the coconut shells are used as fuel and the husks are often used as bristles for cleaning vessels.

In both ayurvedic medicine as well as modern nutrition, coconuts are considered antibacterial, antifungal, antiviral, anti-parasitic, antioxidant, hypoglycemic and hepatoprotective. Coconut flesh consists of various bioactive compounds including vitamin amino acids, organic acids, enzymes and phenolic acids. Coconut water is a refreshing natural drink loaded with antioxidants, anti-inflammatory and immune stimulating effects. Milk extracted from coconut meat is high in a type of saturated fats called medium chain fatty acids. These types of fatty acids are absorbed quickly by our body and used for energy instead of being stored in adipose tissues. Coconut milk has laxative properties as well and has a low glycemic index, which prevents insulin spikes.

More that 1500 studies have been done on coconut to document its various health benefits and studies related with coconut's cancer protective properties have shown positive results.

Peptides isolated from *coconut water* show potential anti-cancer properties. A January 2019 study demonstrated that coconut water vinegar delayed tumor formations and also initiated metastasis of tumor cells (Mohammad *et al*, 2019). It also activates anti-tumor immunity in breast cancer. A compound called dentin ribosome found in *coconut milk* is known to inhibit the growth of multiple myeloma and many other cancers in animal studies (colon, lymphoma, breast etc.) (Ghosh, 2016). Lauric acid makes up 50% of *coconut oil*. Studies show that lauric acid triggers anti-proliferative effects in both breast and endometrial cancer cells. Lauric acid present in virgin coconut oil has shown to release chemo side effects in breast cancer patients. A 2017 study found inhibitory actions of lauric acid in breast cancer, colon cancer and endometrial cancer cells (Lappano *et al*, 2017).

In our practice we have found that the use of coconut water, milk, and coconut oil helps in combating various side effects of chemo and radiation, as well as helping to improve the overall health of cancer patients.

The Cancer Fighting Indian Kitchen

You should consider your kitchen as a Pharmacy or Culinary Pharmacy. A majority of the items should come from a farm and not a factory!

The Pantry

The pantry, better known as a storeroom in Indian households, was traditionally the room or area near the kitchen where items not needed for everyday cooking were kept. It was a place for staples such as grains, rice, and pulses bought in bulk or carried in from one's hometown. Locked with a padlock, the women of the house would have its key tied to the *pallu* of their sarees. Seasonal foods that were dried in the sun, such as *papads* and chilies, were stored there, while in larger homes so were snacks, both sweet and savory, that were prepared in large batches. Rationing food was necessary in homes with sizeable families. If one child finished a week's worth of *laddoos*, there would be no more for the other children of the home!

Today, particularly in the cities, large families are rare, as is the rationing of *laddoos*. These days, food rationing is needed for other reasons, primarily for the control of junk food consumption. Unhealthy foods such as biscuits, chips, chocolates, and samosas are available in

What are real foods?

Nature has a Bounty of foods on her platter to offer. The wide variety of fruits, vegetables, whole grains, legumes, nuts, oilseeds, milk, eggs, seafood and free meat are all considered real foods. Prior to the industrial revolution, majority of our staple diet constituted of these real foods. Our forefathers had access only to locally available foods, making for little variety in food choices (for example, people in coastal region, had fish almost daily). Today we are spoilt for choices. More than half of the food on our platter is either unreal or have been stripped of its nutrients. The polished grains, processed meat products, highly refined oils and hormone laced milk products of today's world cannot be termed real foods.

plentiful quantities and have become the go-to snack for adults and children. Supersized packs of biscuits, instant noodles, and cold drinks are the kind of foods people are buying in bulk these days.

We suggest, instead, to create a cancer-fighting pantry. So, what should you stock it with?

• Store the kinds of staples you regularly eat, whether it be rice, dals, wheat, jowar, or ragi, and other pulses and spices. This is for convenience, so you need not run to the grocers for everyday items.

• Store locally available millets and millet flour

• Tamarind, *kokum*, chilies, dried *amla*, jaggery, oil seeds, nuts, and dried herbs.

• Good quality spices, especially turmeric, *dhania* powder, and *jeera* powder.

- Traditional masala combos; certain communities and some families have their own.
- Dried fenugreek leaves, basil, moringa powder, grated and sundried *amla*, and masalas, both homemade and store-bought.
- Apple cider vinegar, traditional healthy pickles such as lemon pickles, fresh turmeric pickles, and traditional chutneys.
- Homemade snacks.
- And here are some things that should <u>not</u> be in your pantry:
- Try and avoid buying foods in bulk. Sometimes staples need to be purchased this way, but avoid having too many foods in large quantities, as there is too much maintenance required to keep the foods fresh and insect-free.
- There should be no store-bought cookies or wafers. Snacks should not need to be stored for very long. Biscuits like Bourbon, Parle-G, and the like, as well as chips such as Lays potato chips, are junk foods that used to come in small packets and, therefore, rarely eaten in excess. These same foods are now available in giant quantities like in the West, disregarding portion control and adding to the intake of junk calories.

> *Chilli peppers slow down cancer metastasis*
>
> *Researchers have observed that capsaicin in chill peppers (shimla mirchi, mirchi) inhibited the spread of lung cancer cells by suppressing activation of the Protein SRC.*

The Fridge

Your kitchen shelves and refrigerator should not be filled to the brim. Your kitchen should contain as little food as possible, mainly because most of your foods should be fresh fruits and vegetables purchased regularly and consumed quickly. This is not such an issue in India where

Avoid mercury poisoning toxicity from seafood
High Amounts of mercury in some seafood is a big health concern. Seafood is considered to be one the best animal foods and is consumed all over India, especially in the coastal areas. Fish is heart protective, brain protective and the Omega-3 reduces inflammation in the body. However, to protect yourself from mercury toxicity, opt for smaller fish which are less likely to have mercury. Suggested options are golden anchovies (mandeli) Indian mackerel (bangda) Indian salmon (rawas), Bombay duck (bombil), hilsa, pomfret, shrimps, clams, and crab.

fruit and vegetable vendors are on every corner, and many deliver to homes. Unlike the West, which has a colder climate, our refrigerators must work hard to keep things cool. Vegetables wilt and perish much faster in India than abroad. The fresher the vegetable is, the more nutrients it has, so it pays to keep veggies as fresh as possible. Buy or order them regularly rather than buying in bulk. Buy local produce whenever possible.

You can stock your fridge with the following:

•   Fresh herbs such as coriander, mint, and curry leaves can be stored for longer since they are used in small quantities.

- Dried fruits and nuts are healthy snacks that can be stored in your fridge.
- Eggs, hummus, coconut milk, and peanut butter can be included.
- The freezer is a better way to store cooked food longer. You can make large batches of food and store a few servings to eat later. Freshly scraped coconut is regularly stored in the freezer. Whenever

you need it for cooking, it is easily accessible.

- Masalas you do not use frequently.
- Make sure to toss everything that is stale or dated.

Ayurvedic Eating

"One who has all doshas – agni, dhatu, mala – *in a balanced state is considered healthy. Such a person is always happy and content in body, mind and soul."*

– *Shushrut*

Ayurveda is not just the science of healing but also strongly preaches preventive medicine or *swasthavritta* and a healthy lifestyle. Ayurveda offers sound eating principles for overall health, and it is these principles we need to re-inculcate into our food culture:

- Eat whole foods
- Eat local, especially fruits and vegetables
- Eat only when you are hungry
- Do not overeat
- Be mindful when you are eating
- Eat at regular times
- Eat in a comfortable and calm place
- Eat the right quantity
- Eat slowly, chewing your food well

This may seem like a lot of rules, but it is how we used to eat in India — a wholesome home *thali* at regulated times, eaten slowly with attentiveness.

This ancient science believes that digestion (*jathragni*) is the sole basis of health or ill health of a person. In other words, all illnesses stem from the gut. If your eating habits and digestive capabilities are balanced, you can overcome complicated and chronic diseases. In short, Ayurveda strongly advocates working on enhancing our digestive powers.

The most important tenets of this Ayurveda application are:

- Eating only after digestion of prior meals

  Ayurveda believes that only when our body clearly indicates that the prior meal has been completely digested can we consider eating again. The *shloka* (verse) below explains that after the digestion of meals, there is a feeling of energy in both the body and mind.

- Eating to one's constitution (*prakruti*)

  Ayurvedic teachings recognize three *doshas* (biological energies) or *prakrutis,* which derive from the five elements and their related properties: *Vata* is composed of Space and Air, *Pitta* of Fire and Water, and *Kapha* of Earth and Water. Ayurvedic science reveals that a *vata prakruti* person has a low appetite, a *pitta* person has a very high appetite, while *kapha* type's appetite is balanced.

- Eating according to the changing seasons (*rutucharya*)

  Ayurvedic texts mention 6 seasons in a year. The type of food, amount of food, and amount of water are all adjusted according to these seasons.

- Following all the rules and etiquette of eating

  The most important rule Ayurveda advocates is calorie restriction.

  Ayurveda believes that six tastes are essential for a balanced meal and body. Here are some examples of ingredients that embody these tastes across the plate worldwide:

- **Sweet:** whole grains, dairy products, fruits like mangoes, peaches, apricots, vegetables like yams, pumpkin, avocados, and nuts like almonds and cashews.
- **Sour:** yogurt, sour cream, buttermilk, all citrus fruits, tomatoes, strawberries.
- **Salty:** sea salt, soy sauce, olives, mustard, pickles.
- **Pungent:** peppers, ginger, garlic, asafetida, wasabi, horseradish, cumin, cloves.

- **Bitter:** coffee, dark chocolate, brinjal, sesame, bitter gourd.
- **Astringent:** tea, turmeric, grapes, green bananas, basil, rosemary.

"Eat a balance of all six tastes: sweet, sour, salty, bitter, pungent, astringent. If foods of only one taste are eaten, it leads to weakness. If one has a variety of foods including all six tastes, it gives strength and health."

– Charaksamita

[The above *shloka* says that only a person who eats the right foods and eats less can be considered a healthy person. Other rules of eating are eating local foods, eating a wide variety of foods, and not eating stale foods.]

It is important to note here that we are not advocating practicing a full Ayurvedic diet according to your *doshas*. Following these strict rules is not easy in today's times. It is difficult, for example, to strictly avoid certain foods or cook foods differently for all family members' needs. The above rules, however, are doable and should be practiced as much as possible.

> *There are no super foods. There are no miracle foods. Miracles happen when you make a consistent effort in combining all that is good for your health. Miracles happen when you apply the MNM Principle.*

Movement is Medicine!

Exercise is a wonder drug: it reduces your risk of cancer, heart disease, Alzheimer's, diabetes, among other diseases. It lowers cancer risk by helping control weight and insulin levels, strengthens the immune system, and can greatly improve quality of life during cancer treatment as well. Researchers at the American Cancer Society and the National Cancer Institute have confirmed the link between exercise and a lower risk of thirteen specific types of cancer. Their study found that even leisure-time physical activity was associated with a significantly decreased risk of colon, breast, endometrial, kidney cancer, liver cancer, stomach cancer, esophageal cancer, myeloid leukemia, multiple myeloma (blood cancer), and cancers of the head and neck, rectum, bladder, and lungs.

An additional study that was facilitated by the National Cancer Institute in the US over an 11-year period found the following averages in participants with the highest and most consistent level of exercise:

- Breast cancer – risk factor lowered by 10%
- Bladder cancer – risk factor lowered by 13%
- Head and neck cancer – risk factor lowered by 15%
- Colon cancer – risk factor lowered by 16%
- Kidney cancer – risk factor lowered by 23%
- Myeloid leukemia – risk factor lowered by 20%

- Endometrial cancer – risk factor lowered by 21%
- Stomach cancer – risk factor lowered by 22%
- Lung cancer – risk factor lowered by 26%
- Liver cancer – risk factor lowered by 27%
- Esophageal cancer – risk factor lowered by 42%
- Rectal cancer – risk factor lowered by 13%
- Myeloma – risk factor lowered by 17%

Sitting for long periods, whether in front of your laptop at work or the television at home puts you more at risk of cardiovascular disease, diabetes, and cancer. Inactivity causes slow metabolism, which is your body's ability to burn calories. The current fad of using standing desks does not actually help; only walking or movement can increase your metabolic rate, and standing in one place does not achieve this. Fidgeting in place is a better way to increase metabolism than standing desks. The facts are convincing, but fear of disease should not be the reason to move.

> *Try this experiment:*
> *On days that you exercise, do you notice that you have more energy, are in a better mood, and want to talk to people rather than staying in your shell? Exercise elevates your mood; it is the best anti-depressant nature has to offer. We are just not meant to stay sitting for too long.*

Simply put — exercise makes you feel good.

Physical activity is any movement that uses skeletal muscles and requires more energy than resting. This includes working, exercising, household chores, and leisure activities such as walking, trekking, swimming, gardening, and bicycling.

The directive in this principle is movement and not exercise. Movement is a lifestyle, not an event, which means we need to find ways to move in our daily lives. The lifestyle of modern-day middle-class Indians has become fairly sedentary. Household help is relatively inexpensive, and the middle class in India can afford someone to garden, clean, cook, drive, do household repairs, and pick up grocery bags. Air pollution and crowded footpaths in cities and towns also make walking unpleasant.

So, what's to be done? Visiting one of the many gyms and fitness centers that have burgeoned recently is a step in the right direction, but incorporating movement into your daily life is even more important. How can you do this? At work, take hourly bathroom breaks or get up and get some water to drink – put a timer on your phone, if necessary. Do not keep a water bottle on your desk. Make sure you get up and move to get your drink. You will find yourself both refreshed and more productive. The same goes if you are at home. Get up and move as much as possible – if the doorbell rings, get up and answer it yourself, make your bed, clean your closet. Don't be afraid if the help doesn't show up that day; better yet, give your help a day off once a week. Take the stairs instead of the elevator, and walk wherever possible – anything that will get you moving.

We have used the word movement here because the word exercise does not always have a good connotation; it can carry an aura of a burdensome task. In fact, the word originally meant the condition of being in active operation, practice for the sake of training. The original definition likely was applied to the act of driving farm animals to the field to plow – a disciplinary task. Movement, on the other hand, connotes joy. When we get good news, we jump up and down spontaneously. Kids also run and jump when they play. The general idea is to pair the idea of movement with fun.

"Every human being is the author of his own health or disease."
– Gautama Buddha

Part II

The Indian Tools
If Cancer Happens

कालार्थकर्मणां योगा हीनमिथ्याऽ तिमात्रका: ।
सम्ययोगश्च विन्तेयो रोगरोग्यैककारणम् ॥

वाग्भट

*Any physical, verbal or mental work
done in a less, excess, or wrong way leads
to formation of Disease.*

Vag-bhatt
(Ashtang Hridyam)

The word Cancer is often associated with death. However, this is no longer the case. There are so many new developments in Cancer treatments. Patients are living longer and having a better quality of life. In years past, patients would experience nausea, hair loss, and extreme irritation to the intestinal tract no matter what treatments they took, but now there are many chemotherapy treatments that don't cause hair loss or even much sickness. Every year there's more and more research in addition to breakthroughs in treatments and technology.

When side effects do occur, there are ways to mitigate their impact. Understanding your symptoms and finding ways to soothe them as far as possible is crucial, as is keeping a positive attitude. Again, remember, a cancer diagnosis is not a death sentence. You just need to get your body ready to fight the disease.

♦♦♦

Chapter **7** — Hygiene and Kitchen Tips

Hygiene and Kitchen Tips

"One who maintains cleanliness keeps away diseases."

– Sam Veda

The body's immune system is repressed when you go through chemotherapy and/or radiation. The blood cells that protect us against disease and germs are affected and cannot fight infections like before since you are immunosuppressed, and which is why you need to stay away from people who are ill during treatment. The body also cannot fight food-borne illnesses caused by food containing harmful bacteria, parasites, or viruses.

Some foods have a higher risk of becoming tainted with bacteria and should be avoided during treatment. If you cannot live without these foods, be extremely careful when cleaning and preparing them. You and the person helping you take care of your health need to take precautions to avoid possible infection-causing germs.

Here are some tips on how to maintain the utmost hygiene:
- Wash your hands with soapy water before and after preparing food and before eating.

- Keep hot foods hot (warmer than 60°C) and cold foods cold (cooler than 4°C).
- Wash fruits and vegetables well under running water before peeling or cutting. There is no need to use any type of commercial produce rinses. Use a clean scrubber or brush on items that have thick, rough skin or rind (melons, potatoes, bananas, etc.) or any items that have dirt on them.
- Do not share food that is being eaten. There is no English equivalent of the Hindi word *jootha*, which means sharing food while being eaten, but this is a big no-no while on cancer treatment. Our mouths house some of the fastest-dividing cells in the body, making them susceptible to disease. Lots of bacteria are transferred when you take a lick of ice cream from another person's ice cream cone, leaving you open to catching viruses from even that little lick.
- Use different spoons for stirring foods and tasting them while cooking. Do not taste the food with any spoon that will be put back into the food. Do not let anyone else taste the food either. Again, no *jootha*!
- Refrigerate food promptly. Refrigerate or freeze perishable food within 2 hours of cooking or buying it. Proper cooking destroys bacteria, but they can still grow on cooked food that is left out too long, especially in warmer weather.
- Do not cross-contaminate foods. Use a separate clean knife to cut each different kind of food. Always use a different cutting board and knife for raw meats.
- When you thaw meat or poultry, ensure the drippings do not contaminate other areas of the fridge or countertop. Use a dish to catch drips. Do not thaw at room temperature.
- Use defrosted foods right away after thawing. Do not refreeze defrosted food.

Avoid the following:

- Try and avoid raw salad, but if you crave it, clean and cut the salad vegetables thoroughly. Peel carrots, cucumbers, and beets. Unwashed vegetables, especially leafy vegetables, can hide dirt and other contaminants
- Raw sprouts. It is better to sprout them at home and steam them rather than eat them raw. Cooked sprouts are more digestible.
- Choose fruits wisely. You can eat bananas since they have thick, protective skin. Apples and pears washed well and peeled are also okay. Avoid most other thin-skinned fruits, especially berries, grapes, and guava.
- Drink fresh fruit juices only if they are homemade. Homemade orange, sweet lime, and watermelon are allowed if made with excellent hygiene. No fresh juice bought at a restaurant is recommended.
- Raw or undercooked fish, seafood, or meat of any kind.
- Unpasteurized milk. Always boil milk.
- Soft cheeses made from unpasteurized milk, such as brie, camembert, feta, and goat cheese.
- Undercooked eggs, such as soft-boiled and poached, or foods made with raw egg, such as homemade mayonnaise. Throw away eggs with cracked shells.
- Frozen foods, unless you know how they have been frozen. Our Indian cold storage system is sometimes unreliable, and foods often get thawed and frozen again during the distribution network. It is better to avoid these foods.

Cooking Tips:

- Cook foods well.
- Cook meat until it's no longer pink and the juices run clear. If you have a food thermometer, you can check that cooked meat's

internal temperature reaches 70°C and poultry to 80°C. However, it is not necessary to purchase one.

- Minimize the use of plastic containers and never use plastics when heating foods in the microwave. Plastic containers may leach chemicals into the food while being heated at high heat. Use glass containers when re-heating in the microwave.
- Never heat or store food in plastic containers that were not intended for food.
- Let food cool before putting it in a plastic container, then immediately put it in the fridge. Avoid plastics that are stained or damaged or have an unpleasant smell.
- If you buy frozen or refrigerated foods, make sure you place them in your fridge as soon as possible. You should not eat these foods frequently as refrigeration is not reliable in India due to electricity fluctuations.

It might seem like these tips are creating a lot of work for you or your caretaker, but getting food-borne illness during cancer treatment can have a negative impact on the treatment's effectiveness. Prevention is key.

The Role of Nutrition During Treatment

No one can predict how cancer treatment will affect you. Not everyone gets side effects, and for those who do, not everyone has the same side effects or reacts to treatment protocols the same way. Each body responds differently. Some people get absolutely no side effects and have normal appetites throughout treatment; others have days of no appetite, nausea, and diarrhea. For some, side effects decrease or increase over time; for some, they come and go. Most oncologists in India do not believe diet plays a significant role in cancer treatment and do not place much emphasis on patients' food intake. And rightly so. Doctors have your life in their hands and will use the most powerful weapons available to them, which means oncological drugs. Food cannot be a substitute for cancer drugs. Food can, however, play an important role in your body's ability to handle the hit it takes from these toxic therapies. To be clear, toxic does not have a bad connotation here. Toxic medication is what is needed to fight cancer cells. However, these same drugs also attack healthy cells, and this is where nutrition and other healing techniques need to be brought onto the battlefield to fight cancer.

Chemotherapy drugs have improved drastically over time, and the side effects they cause have also been reduced, but their toxicity still takes a toll by attacking the good cells in the body while doing their job of getting rid of the cancerous cells. To be better equipped to handle this, your nutrition will play a role.

People with cancer have unique nutritional needs and issues related to food intake, and these needs keep changing. Most patients with cancer suffer from nutritional deficits, and up to 85% of patients with certain cancer types experience some form of weight loss or malnutrition during cancer treatment.

For some patients, nutritional deficiencies can lead to cancer cachexia, a specific form of malnutrition characterized by muscle wasting, loss of lean body mass, and impaired immune, physical, and mental function. Poor nutrition and weight loss can lead to deteriorating health for patients, with decreased quality of life and increased complication rates with treatment disruptions. Luckily, ensuring good nutrition from the early stages can help patients maintain body weight and lean body mass, enabling them to tolerate treatment better and improve their quality of life.

Appetite may change periodically, and food may taste and smell differently; foods you once loved you may detest, and vice versa. Cancer treatment can also cause nausea, diarrhea, vomiting, constipation, mouth sores, and swallowing problems. These issues may result in weight loss, leading to weakness and fatigue. Some medications may also cause weight gain. Weight gain is not healthy if it makes you overweight. The higher a patient's BMI (Body Mass Index), the greater the chance the cancer will relapse. This is not to scare you; one should not go on drastic diets when undergoing cancer treatment. Likewise, you should not think that gaining weight is healthy. To learn how to calculate your BMI and to understand what a healthy BMI is, please see the FAQs.

The food we eat goes into all our body's cells, and cancer, most simply put, is cells in a state of disease. Doesn't it make sense that we should be feeding these cells well? Good nutrition will also help you recover well and reduce your chances of relapse. Good physical health leads to better mental health, and an improved mental and emotional state helps keep you positive. A positive attitude has been shown to help cancer treatment outcomes.

Several studies have proven that sugar, refined flours, trans fats, and red meats are harmful to health, especially when the body's defense mechanisms are weak and fighting both the disease of cancer and the effects of chemotherapy and radiation. Telling patients not

> *Regardless of the side effects, you may experience, nutrition is an essential part of dealing with cancer treatment. During treatment, you will be using all your energy to combat the disease. Eating well will give you strength and supply you with the nutrients your body needs. Getting the right nutrients will make you stronger as well as feel better.*

to eat sugar, meat, samosas, cakes, and pastries for the months of their treatment protocol has its hazards. This suggested change makes many patients, already dealing with the shock of the cancer diagnosis, feel even more out of control and despondent. The mind-body connection is strong here, so we tell them the dangers of these foods and the fact that it is better to avoid them, but they can have them occasionally in moderation. To restrict something completely does not work, but education about the dangers of certain foods is essential.

There are no hard and fast rules about eating during cancer treatment, but the importance of eating as healthily as possible cannot be overemphasized. Fruits, vegetables, and whole grains should make up the bulk of your calories. Try and eat various foods to get a range of nutrients to stay strong and combat the disease. Use the 80-20 rule as a guideline: as long as 80% of your intake is healthy, you can go ahead and have some of the not-so-healthy foods you may be craving the remaining 20% of the time.

Do not be hard on yourself if there are days you cannot eat due to nausea or lack of appetite. If you are unable to eat at all, then getting any calories is critical. For example, we do not advocate bread consumption, as it is difficult to get good quality bread easily in India, but in this case, the calories are important, and bread is okay. When you have cancer, there is a war going on in your body against the cancer cells, and all is fair in war. If you are having problems eating, talk to your oncology team, as there are many ready remedies and solutions for side effects. The side effects may not go away completely, but you will get some relief.

Case Study

As dieticians, we advocate gradual changes in diet and lifestyle in order to make long-term impacts on health and nutritional goals. Accordingly, the first questions we ask our patients are about their lifestyle and social habits, as both are important determinants of their weight and health.

Mr. Patil was only 30 years old when he came for a weight loss consultation. Late night partying, heavy drinking and smoking caused bouts of acidity off and on for Mr. Patil, resulting in GERD (gastro-esophageal reflux disease). Heartburn and chest pain were his GERD symptoms, but they did not deter him from his partying; he just kept popping antacids and visiting for diet consultation at the insistence of his worried wife. He was monitored for approximately an 18-month period, after which his endoscopy showed Barret's esophagus, which is the narrowing of the food pipe and potentially pre-cancerous. He was warned that he needed to reduce his late nights and drinking, or his condition could worsen. Upon receiving this advice, he did not return to the clinic. Sadly, he succumbed to cancer of the esophagus two years later. The prognosis for esophagus cancer in a young person, such as Mr.

Patil, is fairly good if caught early and certain dietary actions are taken. Mr. Patil did not follow any dietary guidelines even after learning of his pre-cancer diagnosis.

Unfortunately, this is not a one-off case. We have seen habits such as smoking, drinking, overeating, and inactivity cause a host of diseases in a younger and younger population. And even after diagnosis, many individuals are not ready to change their habits. Instead, they look for quick fixes such as antacids and laxatives, making overcoming their ailment more difficult, if not impossible, to achieve.

Healthiest Way to Cook Sabjis

Before you ask the question, what's the healthiest way to cook *sabjis*, first ask yourself if there are enough *sabjis* on your *thali*. As mentioned before, your plate should comprise of 50% vegetables. It is important to have your *thali* half full of vegetables as they are lower in carbohydrates and fat, full of fiber, and give you the highest amount of nutrients. Get accustomed to planning your meals in this way first. After achieving this, extracting more nutrients from your daily *sabjis* is the next step.

You should be making your sabjis with less oil and less cooking time. Oil adds too many calories to your meal. It is a common misconception that the more oil used, the tastier the dish becomes.

For the type of *sabjis* we eat regularly, a teaspoon of oil is enough for a *tadka*. Cook your vegetables on a low flame so they do not need the extra oil for cooking.

As a general rule, steaming is one of the best ways to cook most vegetables. For nutrient preservation, it's best to keep cooking time, temperature, and the amount of water to a minimum, however, traditional steaming won't work with our *sabjis*.

We can achieve the same results by adding minimal water to vegetables after they have been added to the pan following the *tadka*. Adding water to vegetables slowly as needed is also an effective technique to preserve nutrients, provided the veggies are not overcooked. Overcooking results in the loss of important nutrients, which will also drain the flavor. Put a lid on the vegetables and again, cook on a low flame.

List of Indian Sabzis for Cancer Prevention and Post-Cancer Treatment

- Simla Mirchi
- Dal Palak, Aloo Palak
- Potato + Cauliflower
- Cauliflower + Green peas
- Cabbage + Green peas
- Cabbage + Potato
- Green Tomato Sabzi
- Red Tomato Sabzi
- All green vegetables (Methi, Palak, Green onion Amarnath)
- All combinations of Brinjal
- All Beans (French, Drumsticks, etc.)
- All Sprouts Sabzi
- Rajma
- Chickpea curry (Chole)
- Mushroom
- Elephant yam (Suran)
- Pumpkin
- Kohlabi (*navalkon*)
- Okra (*bhindi*)
- All types of Gourds – bitter gourd, bottle gourd, snake gourd, sponge gourd

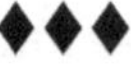

Managing the Side-Effects of Treatment

"Cancer is common now, survival rates are high, but undergoing chemotherapy is still an unpleasant experience."

– Anonymous

Our patients ask us daily what they should eat while undergoing treatment, and if food can help mitigate side effects. The answer, of course, is yes.

The fact is that everything you eat and drink, changes the chemistry of your blood. If you have been eating unhealthy foods, then this will have an adverse impact, and vice versa.

Being proactive with your health through optimal diets and exercise can help inhibit malignant growth, reduce treatment toxicity, improve quality of life, and promote survivorship. For example, breast cancer patients who keep their insulin levels under control through diet and lifestyle cut their risk of cancer recurrence by half and decrease mortality by two-thirds.

Malnutrition created by the inability to eat is a concern for most cancer patients. If patients are too weak due to weight loss from an inability to eat, they may not be able to undergo surgery or chemotherapy required for their treatment. Managing side effects is crucial to your overall treatment.

Eating a plant-based diet consisting of foods on our basic *thali* is fundamental to your cancer battle. Unfortunately, no one likes to feel that they are going on a "diet," especially when ill. Additionally, food can be a solace when you are ill and recovering from treatment. If that is the case, there are plenty of ways to make your *thali* welcoming, interesting, and diverse.

Each body reacts differently to treatment. Some have a difficult time with food intake, while others do not. Some have severe side effects, while others have mild ones. Today, advances in cancer care have led to improved chemotherapy drugs with much fewer side effects, yet these treatments do still affect the lining of the intestinal tract. The following sections detail how to best mitigate the side effects of chemotherapy and radiation with our native foods.

Dry Mouth and Difficulty Swallowing

Many patients experience dry mouth during treatment, making chewing and swallowing difficult. Chemotherapy, anti-nausea medication, radiation, and surgery to the neck region can cause temporary damage to the saliva glands.

Saliva keeps the mouth clean, and its absence creates a breeding ground for bacteria, promoting tooth decay and causing infections. Digestion begins in the mouth with your teeth and gums. When they are painful or diseased, getting the nutrition you need becomes difficult. The tissues of the mouth, gums, and throat are susceptible to soreness during treatment and, optimally, should be in good condition from the onset of treatment. Oral hygiene is imperative to prevent or at least minimize pain when the immune system is depressed from cancer drugs. It is important to see a dentist before your cancer treatment protocol begins to prepare your mouth to cope with infections that can hinder your body's ability to get better.

Here are some tips to employ before meals and during meals:

- Sour tastes often stimulate salivary flow. Ingesting a combination of amla powder and honey throughout the day will increase saliva flow.
- Drink a cup (80-100ml) of fresh lime water 10-15 minutes before beginning your meal.
- Eat smaller, more frequent meals, instead of 3 large ones.
- Avoid dry foods such as toast, *khakra* and *chivada*.
- Avoid sticky foods such as nut butter or *chikki*.
- Take small sips of water while you are eating as this will help you swallow.
- Cold food and drinks may be soothing to the mouth.
- Make food moister. Soak your roti in dal, or add thin curds to your rice, for example.
- Having fresh, homemade pickles that are not too spicy work well to stimulate the saliva. Lemon pickle is an excellent choice.
- Taking small bites and chewing well will make swallowing easier.
- Keep your caloric intake high with protein smoothies and meal replacements.

Tips to try between meals:

- Sip water or ice chips throughout the day. Always keep a water bottle by your side.
- Since bacteria grow rapidly in the mouth and cause tissue infections, it is important to keep the mouth clean. Keep your teeth and tongue brushed and your gums flossed.
- Avoid mouthwashes that contain alcohol, as they can irritate tissues. Instead, you can try homemade mouthwash recipes mentioned in Appendix II at the end of the book.

Soups

Soups are wonderful foods to eat during treatment. They are especially ideal for patients who are having difficulty chewing, swallowing, or digesting whole foods. Using homemade broth or stock for soups is not common in Indian soup recipes; instead, Maggi soup cubes are often used. Although tasty, they contain high amounts of sodium and preservatives. Homemade broth adds flavor to soup without the preservatives and sodium of flavoring cubes and is high in beneficial nutrients.

Flossing is not too common among our population, but it should be, as it is necessary to keep your teeth and gums healthy. You can buy affordable floss at any medical shop or online. Make flossing a habit after brushing your teeth, either in the morning or night.

Varieties of soup broth include vegetables, chicken, mutton, and fish. Each is made by simmering various ingredients, straining off the solids, and saving the liquid broth. Vegetable broth, for example, may contain carrots, onions, garlic, celery, or broccoli. A meat-based broth typically has seasonings, onions, meat bones, and meat. You may refer to the Vegetable Broth recipe in the Appendix.

Oil Pulling

Oil pulling is the practice of swishing or holding oils in the mouth for a certain period of time and then spitting it out. It has been mentioned in ancient Ayurveda texts as swishing (*kawal dharan*) and holding oil (*gandusha*), and its purpose is to get rid of oil-soluble toxins in the body. In Ayurvedic texts, the recommended oil is sesame oil. But in today's world, the most commonly used oils are coconut oil (blended with sesame oil), olive oil, or sunflower oil.

The primary benefit of oil pulling is detoxifying and strengthening teeth and gums. Some holistic practitioners claim the therapeutic effects of oil pulling in cancer, but we do not recommend it to be used as a therapy. In our practices, we have used *kawal dharan* for:

- Removing dryness of mouth (post-radiation)
- Reducing metallic taste (post-chemo)
- Reducing symptoms like the absence of taste, decreased saliva production, nausea, and some dental issues.

Since oil pulling is not a palatable method for anyone, let alone cancer patients, here are some alternative formulas to use in place of oil (swish in the mouth for 2-3 minutes and spit it out):

- Cold Water + honey + sesame oil (for dryness of the mouth)
- Warm water + basil leaves + sesame oil (detox effects)
- Cold water + amla juice + cow's ghee (to remove metallic taste)

Vomiting and Nausea

You may experience nausea or vomiting, or both during your treatment protocol. Chemotherapy and radiation affect the stomach, abdomen, and brain. Ask your doctor about the side effects of the drugs you will receive. If nausea and vomiting are side effects, are there any preventive medications you can take? Nausea is usually easier to prevent than treat. If one anti-nausea medicine is not working, the doctors may prescribe another. If your doctor has prescribed anti-nausea medication, take it as directed.

Stress is often overlooked as a cause of nausea. Just thinking about your chemo or radiation sessions can cause butterflies in your stomach. For some, the first sign of stress is an upset stomach or uneasy feeling in the tummy. Be aware of this and combat it with the right foods. If your stress from things like being in a hospital or seeing blood or needles is severe, talk to a counselor for help to overcome it.

If you are vomiting, dehydration can occur. Try taking a few sips of water every few minutes. Sucking on ice or frozen fruit juice is also an option if you can swallow it easily. Black tea, lemon tea, coconut water, and soup are good options. Once clear liquids are tolerated, try easily digestible foods such as *mung khichdi* or curds rice.

Your once favorite foods may no longer be appealing, and food likes and dislikes can change frequently. One day you might like *sabji*, but the next day, you will not be able to stand the smell of it. Experiment with different foods and see what flavors work for you. At this stage, do not be afraid of wasting food.

Here are some tips for managing nausea before treatment:

- Eat a small, light meal or snack before chemotherapy and radiation treatments unless told differently by your medical team.
- Make a mixture of salt and grated ginger and chew on it a few hours before treatment. Take a bite every half hour or one hour.
- If you get stress-induced stomach problems, prepare mentally for the day. Seek help by talking to a counselor, an upbeat friend, or practice any other stress-busting method such as *pranayama*. Learn to breathe deeply and slowly from your abdomen. We tend to forget to breathe during stressful occasions.
- Listen to some soothing music.
- A few hours before treatment, put an acupressure band around your wrist. These bands are used for motion sickness but can also work on this. They are available online.
- Prepare hydration ahead of time – pack electrolytes. Good old coconut water or *nimbu pani* (lemonade) also do the trick.
- If you do the cooking in the household, have that day's meals cooked by someone else so you do not have to smell any food.
- Do not eat your favorite foods when you are nauseous or not feeling well – you will associate them with sickness.

Tips to prevent nausea during and after treatment:

- Keep food in your stomach by eating frequent, small snacks throughout the day (see Chapter 10 for snack ideas).
- Eat and drink slowly.
- Chew thoroughly.
- Try mixing ½ tsp of grated ginger with 2 tsp sugar and ½ lemon. Take it every few hours if it makes you feel better. Both ginger and lemon have anti-nausea properties. Ginger and lemon black tea also helps.
- Grate fresh amla and dry it in the sun by adding some salt. Thee dried amla flakes can be added to fennel seeds (badishep), which helps in combating nausea and dyspepsia.
- Avoid fried, oily and fatty foods. Fat causes food to remain in the stomach longer, increasing the chance of vomiting. Avoid all deep-fried foods, meats, high-fat milk and cheeses, butter, ghee, nut butter such as peanut butter, and bakery products made with fat like pattice and cookies.
- Eat foods that are easy to digest – *khichdi* and curds rice, for example. Have dry foods such as homemade *khakra*, makhana, and whole-wheat toast.
- Avoid drinks with a lot of sugar as they worsen your nausea. If dehydration is an issue, try electrolyte powders. Sugar also remains in the stomach longer and can cause nausea.
- Have dried toast or *khakra* with no oil first thing in the morning or for pre-meal nausea. Toast is a bakery product and not the healthiest option, but it is okay to consume during these times.
- Starchy foods are sometimes helpful when you have nausea: rice, toast, *poha, idlis, bhakris, and murmura.*
- Bland foods may be easier to tolerate such as *makhana.*
- Make mealtimes relaxing. Mealtime conversations should be pleasant. If you are alone, you can read or watch TV (this is contrary

to most advice about not having distractions when eating but is recommended for these circumstances).

- Rest after meals – preferably sitting and not lying down.
- Try and avoid cooking smells. Use an exhaust fan. If someone else is cooking, close the kitchen door, or stay far away from the kitchen area.
- Reduce heavy perfumes, household cleaners, and personal care products with strong smells – any powerful scent can cause nausea.
- Suck on frozen fruit such as watermelon and muskmelon. Just cut up these fruits into bite-sized pieces and put them in a glass container for freezing. Avoid thin-skinned fruits such as grapes and berries.
- Do not take medications on an empty stomach unless directed by the doctor.
- Combat stress with breathing, praying, talking – anything that works for you.
- Position is important. Eat at a table, not in the living room. Do not lie down immediately after eating.
- Clear or salty liquids are easy to keep down. Thin dals, soup, or salted lassis are good options.
- Take care of your oral hygiene – keep your teeth and tongue clean and your mouth rinsed. This will help keep unpleasant odors and bacteria from developing.
- Keep your surroundings fresh and not stuffy; open some windows. Sit on the balcony/terrace/in the garden for fresh air.
- If you are really not up to eating, then take a break. Not eating for a short period will not harm you.
- If you have severe nausea or vomiting and none of the above strategies work, then call your doctor, as you may require IV fluids and nutrition.

Diarrhea

Diarrhea is a common side effect and more annoying than medically distressing. Here are a few do's and don'ts.

Do eat	Do not eat
Starchy foods such as potatoes, rice, whole wheat toast, ripe bananas *upma*, *poha*, and *idli*. Stick to dals that are easy on the stomach, like *moong* and *masoor*; avoid *toor*, *chana*, and *udad* dals.	Hot foods. Hot and warm foods stimulate muscle movement. Try cold foods or foods at room temperature.
High potassium foods to replenish this important electrolyte. Bananas, potatoes, sweet potatoes, and mushrooms are good options.	Milk/dairy. Chemo can cause a temporary absence of lactate, the enzyme that digests lactose (milk sugars).
Homemade *dahi*, preferably with cow's milk. It is a natural source of friendly bacteria and acts as a natural probiotic.	Raw foods as they contain too much fiber.
Nutmeg (*jaayphal*) and mace (*javitri, gala*) are known to help diarrhea. Use mace in your cooking. Grate some nutmeg on your *dahi*.	Very spicy foods such as certain pickles and foods with green chilies

Drink at least 1 cup of liquid after each loose bowel movement.	Certain dishes heavy on spices such as chicken curry, biriyani, veg kolhapuri, etc.
Drink and eat high-sodium (salt) foods like soups and homemade lemon pickle.	Apricots (*jardaloo*), black and yellow raisins, and figs as they have laxative effects.
	Too much coffee and tea.
	Sodas and sports drinks. They contain too much sugar, which can aggravate diarrhea.
	Diet drinks – they have no food value and cannot replace valuable nutrients lost in fluids.
	Foods that cause gas such as beans and certain vegetables in the cabbage family like cabbage, broccoli and cauliflower. These are all very good for you but if your diarrhea is persistent, it is better to choose other vegetables at this time.

Meal suggestions during episodes of diarrhea:
- Curds rice with peeled apple
- Plain *moong khichdi* and clear soup
- Rice *kanji* and peeled apple
- *Rajgeera laddoo* and buttermilk

- Rice pancake (roti/dosa) with mint (*pudina*) chutney and pomegranate
- Peeled apple, orange and clear sop
- Baby formula such as Cerelac with grated apple

Mouth Sores

Mouth sores and sore throats are common side effects of chemotherapy. Good oral hygiene is important and will enable you to manage soreness as well as obtain the nutrition you need. The texture of foods will play an important role here. You may find you like or dislike the feeling of certain foods in your mouth.

Tips:
- Puree foods in the mixer to make them easier to swallow.
- Eat foods cold or lukewarm rather than hot. This will reduce the irritation.
- Avoid spicy food with strong masalas and raw spices.
- Eat soft, bland foods like curds rice, *dahi*, *khichdi*, *idli*, *upma*, dals, puddings, *payasams*, and wheat pasta.
- Avoid dry and coarse foods – use dals and *dahi* to soften the drier items on the *thali*.
- Use a straw to bypass mouth sores. Plastic straws have been banned for a good reason; however, you can purchase steel and paper straws online.
- Eat foods high in protein and calories to help healing.
- Avoid sodas and alcohol.
- Use a mouthwash prescribed by your doctor or a homemade herbal rinse (see Appendix II for homemade mouthwash recipe).

Changes in Taste

Sweet, salty, sour, and bitter are the four taste sensations that are stimulated by your taste buds. These taste buds are formed from fast-dividing epithelial tissue and are particularly sensitive to cancer therapies. Radiation can injure or kill taste buds, and this effect lasts 2-3 weeks after radiation sessions. Infections of the mouth that cause inflammation of the mucous membranes may decrease taste sensations as taste receptor cells become inflamed. These are not life-threatening complications but make getting proper nutrition more difficult as the loss of taste also leads to a loss of appetite. When you have limited taste sensations, make every calorie count.

Tips:

- Do not eat favorite foods during chemo, which may cause an aversion or unpleasant association with the food.
- Suck on a lemon drop, *amla supari*, mint drop, or *imli goli* during the treatment.
- Foods that are cold or at room temperature may be more tolerable than hot ones.
- Unpleasant food smells may get associated with unpleasant tastes – avoid food smells as much as possible.
- Try different *tadkas*, flavorings, and spices, and see if they agree with you.
- Do not use steel vessels for cooking. Instead, try our traditional clay pots, now renamed in the market as earthen cookware.
- Use bamboo spoons instead of steel/metal. The feel and taste of metal may not agree with you. Even better, use your hands – our traditional hygienic way of eating.
- Rinse your mouth thoroughly after eating.
- Hydration is important. If water is unappealing, consider flavoring your water naturally with mint or cucumber.
- Appeal to your other senses – visuals and texture may stimulate appetite.

Constipation

Treatment protocol, medications, decreased physical activity, and stress can all cause constipation during cancer treatment. Radiation and surgery can also cause temporary nerve damage to the colonic muscles.

Here are some suggestions on how to cure or prevent constipation:

- Drink a glass of hot water first thing in the morning.
- Take *Isabgol*. If you do not like drinking it plain, then add it to your food – rotis and dals, for example. Increase water intake to 2 liters a day. Keep 2 bottles filled in the morning so you can see how much you are drinking.
- Increase dietary fiber. Millets and grains like ragi and brown rice have more fiber than the white varieties. Switching it up also helps with constipation.
- Eat raw vegetables (see hygiene section). Chew thoroughly, with small bites. Grate or blend them if chewing is a problem.
- Eat more vegetables in the cabbage family — cabbage, broccoli, and cauliflower. The gas they produce will help increase the volume and ease bowel movements.
- Nuts and seeds are high in fiber. Flaxseed helps with constipation. Make a mild dry chutney with flaxseed and have it with your meals.
- Eat dried apricots, prunes, and manuka – all have laxative effects.
- Reduce or eliminate milk and cheese, as they have constipating effects on some people.
- Drink warm liquids such as warm lemon water with honey before meals to stimulate the gastrointestinal tract.
- Get some exercise. This stimulates the bowels as well. Ask your doctor if this is okay.
- If you're prone to constipation, try to set up a regular plan for bowel movements. This may include an over-the-counter stool softener or

laxative. Talk to your oncologist about what to use.

- Use laxatives only as directed by your doctor.
- Use ayurvedic laxatives such as *isabgol* and *triphala churna*. Triphala is an ayurvedic preparation which is a combination of amla, *hirda* and *behda* (dried form of fruits) that can be safely consumed in tablet or powdered form. Our experience is that although they are milder than allopathic laxatives, they are effective, cause no harm, and are non-habit-forming.
- Try some constipation-relieving yoga poses.

Constipation Do's and Don'ts

Do eat	Do not eat
Ragi, rice, and *rajgeera*.	Millets (jowar, bajra).
Gourd family vegetables – pumpkin, bottle gourd, snake gourd, *ghosale*, etc.	Bean family vegetables (sword beans, cluster beans, etc.)
Ripe bananas, chickoo, mango, orange, kiwi, papaya, watermelon, sweet lime, and pomegranate.	Apple, pear, and guava.
Milk, *dahi*, and cow's ghee.	Buttermilk, mawa, and cheese.
Green leafy vegetables, cruciferous vegetables, and fish.	
Soups, raita, *rasams*, porridges, *kadhi*, and *koshimbir*.	Dry salads.
Dals.	Pulses (except green gram).
Sherbets – lemon and *kokum*.	Cold drinks and excessive coffee and tea.

Rice-based dishes, ragi porridge, *makhana, rajgeera* ladoo, *aloo paratha*, and *dhokla*.	*Bhakri, namkeen, murmura, bhadang*, roasted *chana, futana*, peanuts, *khakra, papad*, pickles, *badishep, chaat*, and bakery products.
Scrambled eggs with spinach.	Egg curry and boiled eggs.
Chicken pulao with mild spices.	Spicy chicken and mutton curries.

Yoga Poses for Constipation

1. *Pavanamuktasana* or the Wind-Relieving Pose – The name itself shows that it is effective for removing gases and improving the digestive system.

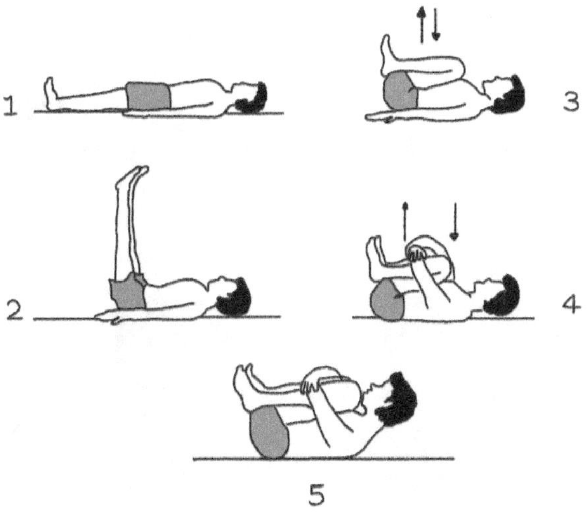

2. *Paschimottanasana*, or the Forward Bending Pose – This deep intra-abdominal compression massages the abdominal viscera. You need to suck in the belly and breathe normally for the pose.

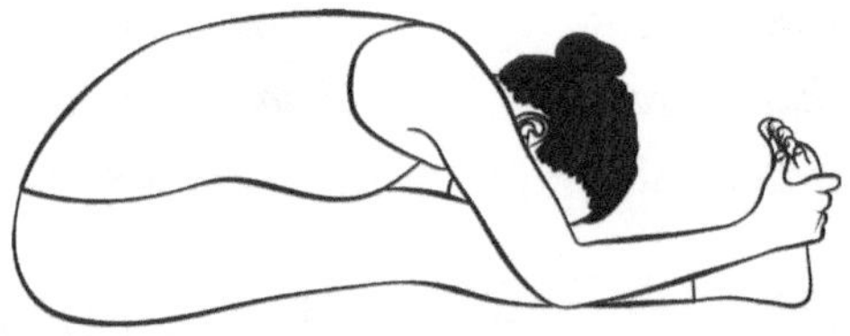

3. *Dhanurasana* or the Bow Pose – This asana strengthens the entire range of abdominal organs. The pressure on the intra-abdominal muscles releases gas and helps with digestion.

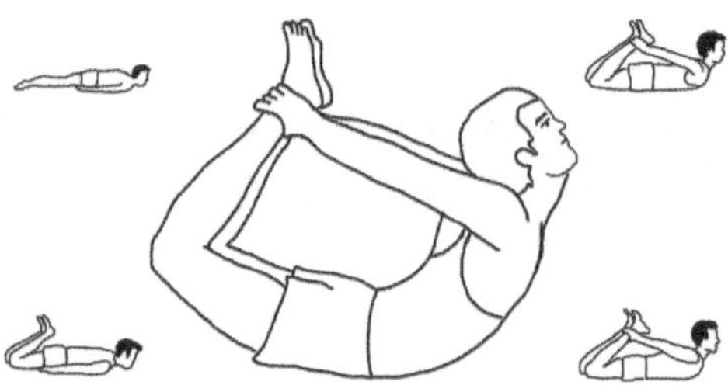

4. *Vajrasana* or The Adamant Pose – This pose improves blood circulation to the abdominal region, helping improve digestion. It is considered one of the best yoga asanas for constipation and indigestion.

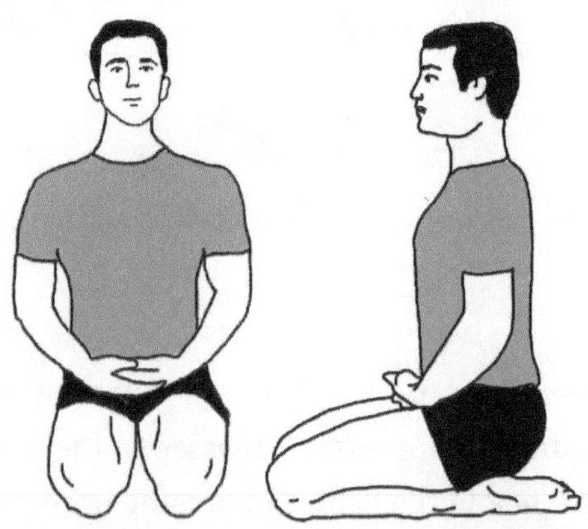

5. *Bhujangasana* or the Cobra Pose – This asana strengthens the abdominal muscles and cleans the entire digestive tract.

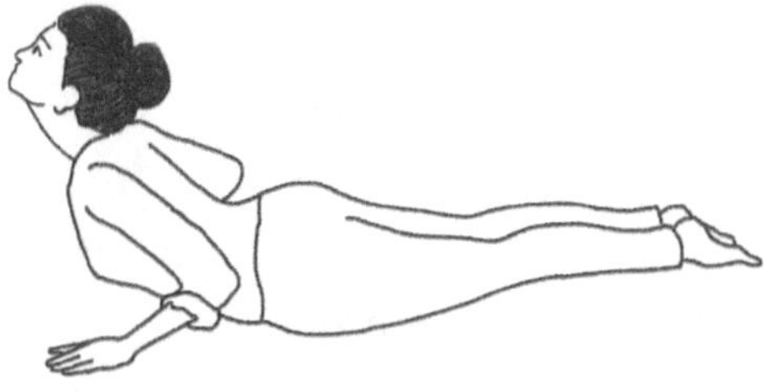

Flatulence and Gas

Flatulence often accompanies diarrhea. Avoiding these foods may help:

- Beans – soy, *moth*, kidney.
- Cruciferous vegetables – cauliflower, cabbage, broccoli
- Onions
- Dairies such as cheese and paneer (*Dahi* and buttermilk are okay)
- Raisins and prunes
- Chewing gum
- Apple juice and carbonated drinks
- Raw salads, carrots, brinjals, spinach, and wheat are mildly gaseous in nature.

Instead, add these foods to your meals:

- Lukewarm water
- Carrom seeds (*ajwain*)
- Cumin seeds
- Black pepper
- Fennel
- Cardamom
- Ginger

The ayurvedic combination called *hingwastak churna* can come handy for gas problems.

Try incorporating these habits for general well-being:

- Eating slowly.
- Sipping water and not gulping it down.
- Not talking while eating.
- Taking a short walk after eating – 100 steps, or *shatapawli*, as it is known, is meant for digesting food.
- Not lying down for at least an hour after eating a meal.

'Chhota Thali': Lighter Meals Throughout the Day

Some side effects (weight loss, diarrhea, nausea) make it difficult to eat an entire *thali*. Eating a *chota thali*, a small quantity several times a day, will be necessary to keep up your strength and mitigate side effects. Splitting up the *thali* and eating more snack-type foods will be a significant part of your daily calorie intake. Small, frequent meals throughout the day may be better to combat side effects and steady your energy levels.

There is no dearth of Indian snacks; many can be made in advance and stored, which will be helpful during treatment. The following is a list of some not-so-usual snacks which may add variety to the palate.

Some healthy snack ideas:
- Watermelon with a few pistachios
- Fresh figs baked in the oven with a dash of honey and nuts of your choice
- Hummus with cut veggies
- Fruit with peanut butter
- Dry Fruits – raisins, dates, apricots, or a medley of them all
- Popcorn or Makhana, flavored with your favorite seasoning: chaat masala, pesto, *jeera*, lime, and chili... the possibilities are endless

- Hard-boiled eggs are very filling, and no toast is needed
- Muesli with *dahi* – something crunchy to go with something creamy
- Buttermilk – add digestives such as *hing* or cumin
- Pickle sandwich – a forgotten, age-old favorite. Put lime pickle on one side of the chapati, and a touch of homemade butter
- Roasted pumpkin seeds
- *Dahi poha* – this is a healthy snack that is often taken on long journeys. Eat half a cup
- Corn *Bhel* – add tomatoes, onions, ginger, garlic, *dhania* leaves, chaat masala, and, voilà, it's ready
- Chocolate with nuts - just a little!
- Masala Oats with veggies
- Roasted seasonal produce – *Hurda* (tender *jowar*) from Maharashtra and *makhana* from Bihar
- Strawberries dipped in chocolate

Our homemade Indian staples are also always good. No book can encompass them all, but here are a few ideas to get you started:

- Indian instant *dosas* such as *pesaruttu* and *rava dosa* from the south of India, *cheela* from the north, and *ghavan* and *amboli* from Maharashtra.
- *Upma* – add veggies like carrots, peas, and tomatoes for a healthier kick
- *Poha* – add veggies like carrots, peas, and tomatoes for a healthier kick
- *Idli upma* – made with leftover *idli*
- *Laddoos*
- *Chakli*
- *Kadboli*

- *Dhokla*
- *Khandvi*
- *Thepla*
- *Thalipith*
- Spicy *chana chaat*
- Vegetable cutlets
- *Rava idli*
- *Paratha*
- Steamed corn (add spices of your choice)
- *Appe*
- Fruit *Chaat*
- *Bhutta*

Post Radiotherapy Soft Diet

At times after radiotherapy treatment, it is difficult to eat solid foods. To enhance caloric content of foods you consume during this time use coconut milk extracted at home or MCT oil. For example, if you are taking ragi porridge or rice porridge add coconut milk or MCT to the porridge.

If you are on a liquid or soft diet, eat small meals every 2 hours, at least 6 meals a day. Ask your oncologist about the use of protein powder and incorporate it regularly in your diet. Proteins and foods with good calories are important tools for protection against post radiation/ chemotherapy weight loss also known as cachexia.

Sample Indian Menus for Cancer Patients

The first sample menu is targeted for the period when you are undergoing cancer treatment but is in-between chemo or radiation days. It may be difficult to follow a proscribed diet during the days of chemo and radiation and a few days after as you may be dealing with side effects.

The next three sample menu is for the time when you are undergoing radiation or chemotherapy. You may be experiencing side effects and will also be immune compromised. Since each individual will experience unique side effects or none at all, comprehensive weekly menu plans do not apply.

Sample Menu 1

(not to be taken during chemotherapy weeks)
These chemo sample diets plans are light on the stomach and contain optimal nutrition.

	Monday	Tuesday	Wednesday	Thursday	Friday
Morning	Lemon/black/green tea OR warm water with ½ lemon				
Mid-morning Breakfast	Rice pancakes with curry leaf chutney	*Pesaruttu* (green moong pancake)	Ragi porridge	*Aloo* pumpkin *paratha* with *pudina* chutney	*Aloo* pumpkin *paratha* with *pudina* chutney

Lunch	Roti with pumpkin *sabji* with *moong dal* and homemade buttermilk	Roti and *palak sabji* with dal and dahi	Roti with green tomato *sabji* with *moong dal*	Roti with *bhindi sabji* and *toor* dal	Ragi roti with *gobi-*potato *sabji* and dal
Afternoon Snack	*Kothimbir* wadi	*Makhana*	*Dhokla*	Dates and nuts	Soup
Dinner	*Mattar* rice with Fresh turmeric pickle	*Moong khichdi* with curry leaf chutney	Mixed veg pulao + beetroot soup	*Moong khichdi* and pudina chutney	Jowar roti with green leafy vegetables and a dal of your choice

Note:

- All foods mentioned above to be homemade.
- Seasonal fruits can replace evening snacks. Fruits are the healthiest snack options, especially if they have thick peels. See pg. xxx for eating fruit). However, chemo weakens the digestive system so if your oncologist has advised you against raw foods then avoid fruits and salads.

Additionally, these diet plans are predominantly alkaline (see Appendix I to know more about alkaline foods) with homemade Indian foods. This works well for pre-chemo, post-chemo, and post-surgery. The meals are digestible and nutritious. The daily protein content is on the lower side – but if your doctor has advised you that higher protein is needed, you should add protein such as dal, pulses, eggs, and fish or supplementary proteins such as protein powder. Alternatively, you can add protein powder to any of the *sabjis*, dals, or *dosa* batters to enhance its nutritional content (see homemade protein powder recipe in Appendix II).

Sample Menu 2
(to be taken during chemotherapy)

	Diet Plan 1	Diet Plan 2	Diet Plan 3
Morning	1 Boiled egg with 5 Overnight Soaked Almonds	Green tea OR ginger tea OR lemon water	Freshly made fruit juice, no added sugar
Breakfast		Rice pancake with mint chutney OR *Tadka* rice with tomato chutney OR *Nagali* (ragi porridge)	Ragi *dosa* with mint chutney
Mid-morning	1 *Rajgeera Laddoo* OR 1 Orange OR 1 Sweet Lime	Coconut Water	Coconut Water OR *Kokum Sherbet*
Lunch	Curds with Rice (as per appetite, the amount can be adjusted)	Curd Rice with baked potato *sabji* and pomegranate OR beetroot juice	Rice pancake with pumpkin *sabji* OR snake gourd *sabji* with buttermilk
Late Evening	Lemon water OR coconut water	*Rajgeera laddoo* OR *Makhana* OR *Ragi* puffs	Soft pulpy fruits like banana, chickoo, papaya, orange, sweet lime, mango – all washed and peeled
Dinner	*Moong dal khichdi* with Mint chutney	*Moong khichdi* with Mixed Veg. Soup OR *Solkadhi* OR Fish Curry	Veg. Pulao cooked with potato, carrots, green peas OR Chicken/Egg Pulao with flaxseed chutney

Note:

Diet Plan 1 is especially beneficial when experiencing weakness and diarrhea. A boiled egg can be replaced with a protein powder prescribed by a doctor or dietician. If you are unable to digest proteins, take ½-1 cup of ready-made baby food powder. This is an easy food shortcut when you lack energy, no inclination to cook, or cannot tolerate the smell of cooked foods.

There may be times during treatment when eating will be difficult. Chemo and radiation may cause nausea, diarrhea, change in taste, and other gastric problems. For the days when you are getting chemo in the hospital or clinic, you can also make a simple porridge so that when you do feel like eating something, food is easily made ready (see Appendix II for the Homemade Porridge Powder recipe).

The following porridge recipe should be kept at hand so. It is also great. You can flavor it with any spices you feel like at the time.

Sample Menu 3

Post Radiation Soft Food Diet Plan Example

Morning	Mid-morning	Lunch	Late Afternoon	Dinner	Late Night
Ragi porridge OR Ragi and Amaranth flour porridge. Add protein powder.	Carrot or red pumpkin pureee OR Ripe papaya paste. Have with soya or coconut milk.	Rice porridge OR Mutton soup OR Rice and Dal Soup OR Overcooked Soft Khichdi. All with added protein powder.	Banana OR Custard Apple OR Papaya paste plus Peanut Butter.	Mashed Sweet Potato with protein powder OR same menu as lunch.	Any type of instant baby food OR pome-gran-ate juice.

A Note for Caregivers

Just like no one wants to be diagnosed with cancer, no one wants to be handed the role of a cancer patient's caregiver. It isn't easy seeing your loved one suffer. Caregivers of cancer patients, usually family members, accompany the patient to the doctor, ask needed questions, and make necessary decisions with the patient and medical care teams. They also significantly influence how the patient deals with their illness. Caregivers are involved in all aspects of the Mind-Nutrition-Movement (MNM) Principle since they keep the spirit and mood of their loved ones positive, feed them healthy, nourishing food, and encourage them to get exercise during treatment. It is a full-time occupation.

In terms of nutrition, if you are a caregiver, you should follow the tips on the side effects of the treatment offered in chapter 9. Consult the oncologist and dietician about any specific diet recommendations. Remember that treatment, especially chemo, can change taste buds, cause nausea, and make food taste metallic.

Do not feel offended or frustrated if you cook food and the patient does not want to eat it. It is common for cancer patients to be fussy in addition to having all the other common side effects. Keep trying and do not lose heart. The nourishment you provide will go a long way and help your loved one gain the strength they need to fight the disease.

Caregiver burnout is a serious issue that also needs to be recognized. Caregiver burnout happens when the caregiver is in a state of distress for a prolonged period and can happen to the strongest and healthiest people. This stress and burnout can affect your health and make you moody, tense, angry, depressed, irritable, or fearful. The fear of the unknown can make you feel lonely, out of control, and unable to concentrate. It is not uncommon to have symptoms such as problems with sleeping, digestion, weight loss or gain, fatigue, frequent colds, and infections – just to name a few!

The following are some tips to help you get through this challenging time:

- Keep nuts handy, especially during long waits at the hospital.
- Pack a protein smoothie as well.
- Keep an eye on your caffeine intake. It feels good to have tea/coffee, which can be a stress buster but can also impact your sleep.
- Get some sleep – have friends help you with the patient as needed.
- Don't feel guilty getting rest; lie down when you need to.
- Get a check-up yourself. Take supplements to keep your immunity and energy levels up.
- Use shortcuts when necessary. Sometimes it may not be possible to prepare an entire *thali* the way you would like.

> *Remember to take care of yourself. Caregiving is physically, mentally, and emotionally taxing. To help your loved one suffering from cancer, it is vital that you are both physically and emotionally fit. The anti-cancer MNM principles are take-aways for you as well.*

Part III

Post-Cancer Management with MNM

अन्नेत पुरयेत अर्धं तोयेन च तृतीयकम्।
उदरस्य तूरीयांश्च संरक्षेत वायुधारणात्॥

घेरंडसंहिता

Imagine your stomach has four equals parts.
Fill half with food, 1/4th with water and leave 1/4 th empty.
Gheranda Samhita

After months or years of undergoing nauseating chemotherapy and radiation, you have achieved your goal of being cancer-free. This is a time to be ecstatic, however this is not always the case, and many patients suddenly feel alone and scared. There are no more regular checkups with the oncologist and the support of family and friends diminishes as you no longer need as much help.

As a cancer patient you have gone through a life-changing experience -- the treatment protocol has taken a toll on you both physically and emotionally. Relapse is always a possibility, an unfortunate stress that is part of the disease.

The principles of MNM at this time are essential to your long-term recovery. Mind, Nutrition and Movement will allow you to manage stress, and get stronger and healthier.

Chapter 13

Mind: Insomnia and Stress Management

Insomnia in Cancer

A restful sleep restores and rebuilds the body's cells and tissues, which is especially important during cancer treatment. Unfortunately, cancer patients are twice as likely to suffer from insomnia, making the healing process even more demanding. Fear of treatment outcomes, financial worries, and anxiety over family responsibilities are common and often cause restless nights.

Maintaining good sleep habits such as sleeping and waking up at regular times, sleeping in cool temperatures, and avoiding caffeine after 4pm are vital. Meditation and pranayama are known to help with sleep, and you should refer to Chapter 1 for more info on these techniques. Just 5-10 minutes of relaxing meditation can help with falling asleep. You should also let your doctor know in case you are facing sleep issues.

Avoid alcohol, spicy food, and caffeine near bedtime, as they affect sleep quality. Some milk (if it does not cause any gastric distress) or a handful of almonds or walnuts are good bedtime snacks if you feel like eating near sleep time; both nuts and dairy contain sleep-promoting agents. Nutmeg is considered an herbal sedative in Ayurveda. Grate half a teaspoon into dairy, almond, or coconut milk and drink it at least two hours before bedtime. You can grate it in a shot of amla juice or plain water as well. Additionally, *tulsi* leaves are believed to have potent powers to flush out toxins from the body and are also used as a natural remedy to reduce anxiety. Use *tulsi* to season your dinner, or drink *tulsi*-flavored water throughout the day. Having something to drink just before bedtime, such as a glass of milk or tea, is not recommended, as it may create an urge to urinate that will wake you from sleep.

It is believed that certain plants emit positive energy, act as natural air purifiers, and can also help improve your sleep. Here are a few of them:

- Aloe Vera: This common plant is quite easy to grow and maintain. It emits O2 during the night.
- Snake Plants: Snake plants are considered one of the best air-purifying houseplants.
- Lavender: Lavender oil is commonly used in aromatherapy and is known to reduce anxiety and stress levels and help you sleep.
- Jasmine: This plant also has soothing effects on our bodies. It is known to reduce anxiety and bring positive energy.
- Spider Plant: This plant absorbs bad odors and is said to cleanse the air of cancer-causing chemicals.

Stress Management

Your support system is also a crucial stress reducer. In India, we have an innate network of family ties, although, with migration to the cities, this scenario is changing somewhat. The city's nuclear families and long work hours make it difficult to foster relationships. For cancer support, we suggest that you nurture your relationships when you have the chance and have gratitude for the people in your life. Support groups attached to your hospital or clinic are also great resources to connect to others.

Adrenaline pours into the body when you stress about the smallest of things. Knowing how to calm the nervous system is essential to healthy living. Some people with cancer say yoga helps calm the mind, allowing them to cope better with their cancer and its treatment. Others say it helps to reduce symptoms and side-effects such as pain, tiredness, sleep problems, and depression. Yoga can also sometimes help you move around more quickly and easily after surgery for cancer. The renowned Dana Farber Cancer Institute in Boston has used yoga as a therapy for over 15 years. Both their adult and pediatric wings offer it as a form of relaxation. A few hospitals in India have incorporated yoga workshops, but overall, there remains a large potential treatment gap that needs to be filled.

Both the diagnosis and treatment of cancer pose physical and psychological threats to the patient. Serious side-effects such as a change in appearance, infertility, altered sexual functioning, hair loss, fatigue, nausea and vomiting, pain, infections, and low blood counts can grossly affect a patient's overall functional quality of life. Moreover, fear and anxiety associated with invasive treatment procedures, sexual dysfunction secondary to surgery and radiation, and aggressive medical treatment are among cancer patients' most common treatment-related side effects. Ironically, while cancer detection and treatment advances have improved survival rates for most cancer patients, surviving cancer means ongoing anxiety about relapse and impending

There are several effective methods of stress-reduction, such as visualization and mindfulness practices. Yoga is especially attractive as it combines many of these techniques with simple stretching exercises, breathing, meditation, and relaxation techniques and nurtures the mind-body connection.

death. This can lead to unwelcome thoughts and feelings of fear, hopelessness, and helplessness, all causing severe psychological distress, which weakens the immune system and reduces the patient's ability to tolerate pain and symptoms.

Results from several studies on yoga and cancer show a positive link and establish the fact that yoga interventions can play a role in the treatment of side-effects of the disease.

Yoga During Treatment

Our bodies are designed to move, and it is important to move as much as possible even when you have cancer (if you don't have pain and with your doctor's approval). Breathing is counted as a movement — your diaphragm does a lot of moving as you breathe. If you cannot do standing yoga postures, gentle movements incorporating breath and meditation techniques are best at this time. You can also do poses that don't require you to leave the floor or your bed: baddakonasna, viparat karni, and ananda balasana are good starting poses and can help with relaxation, anxiety, and sleep.

Yoga After Treatment

After treatment comes remission. The cancer is behind you and is no longer at the forefront of every thought or conversation. However, there is always a feeling of anxiety before the next scan and fear of recurrence. You also may be coping with the side-effects of chemo and radiation long after you have had them. Yoga can play a crucial role here, not only to reduce anxiety but to help take back control of your body. Yoga will help you get mentally and physically stronger and gain confidence to overcome your fears.

Yoga can be transforming during all phases of your cancer journey. For beginners, simple timed inhalations and exhalations are a good start. You can adapt the practice to the needs of your current physical state or stage of treatment. If you're on chemo or have bone metastasis or tumors and are experiencing pain, please don't do anything that hurts. Never push into pain!

Case Study

Leena frequented the clinic for weight loss and chronic obesity problems. She ran a machine parts workshop which demanded quite a bit of travel, leaving less time for exercise. Her hectic schedule also did not allow her to eat at regular times, leading to acidity and hormonal imbalances. Leena's weight was a constant source of anger for her and she was always on the lookout for the latest wellness and diet trends. In 2015, Leena was diagnosed with breast cancer after she noticed a lump in her breast.

Leena decided to take on the disease head on – she studied and researched breast cancer extensively, trying different alternative therapies. All her energy was used in getting rid of the disease but in a way that caused her stress and angst. Her husband and oncologist both told her to slow down but Leena was adamant, "all I want is to get rid of this damn disease and get back to my work."

Leena was technically doing everything right such as eating right and maintaining hygiene. However, she developed many issues during her chemo rounds. Her blood count refused to rise, she caught colds constantly and developed severe unexplained headaches.

Leena came back to my clinic many months later and I noticed a new person. She was actually smiling! She explained to me what had happened over those 8-9 months. When she was the weakest both mentally and physically during her treatment, a relative introduced her to a spiritual group. Leena was resistant at first as she did not believe the science of how this group would help her, but then relented and decided to try it out.

She was first taught to let go of her hatred of cancer. She learned to look at her suffering as an unpleasant experience, which would eventually be a thing of the past. She learned meditation and forgiveness and as time went on, she began responding more favourably towards the chemo treatment.

Today, Leena is not only cancer free but a changed person. She has learned to slow the pace of her life and enjoy the small joys of life. Leena is happy to say that cancer did what no one else could do for her in those years.

Nutrition: Weight Gain, and Weight Loss

Weight Gain

Many people with cancer think they will lose weight and are surprised, and sometimes upset when they end up gaining weight instead. Weight gain can happen for several reasons and certain types of cancer pre-dispose a patient to this outcome. Here are a few:

- Hormone therapy, certain types of chemotherapy, and steroids can cause weight gain. These treatments can also cause your body to retain water, causing bloating.
- Chemotherapy can lead to weight gain in many ways, including edema, which occurs when the body holds on to excess fluid. Edema can cause nausea, which is improved by eating. Chemo can trigger severe food cravings, decrease metabolism, and cause menopause in some women, which also decreases metabolism.
- Steroids cause certain side effects such as an increase in appetite and an increase in fatty tissue (with long-term use), which can increase the size of a person's abdomen, neck, and face. Steroids can cause wasting of the muscles and muscle mass loss. This occurs more frequently in the limbs. Steroids also cause central obesity.
- Hormone therapy is used to treat breast, uterine, prostate, and testicular cancers by decreasing the amount of estrogen or

progesterone in women and testosterone in men. This process can increase fat, decrease muscle, and lower metabolism.

- Cancer treatments can cause fatigue and changes in your daily schedule, which can reduce activity and therefore lower caloric expenditure. In India, the patient is often pampered and not allowed to do housework, which worsens the situation.

- There is also a clear weight gain cause and effect from the Indian diet. The concept of adding rich, fatty ghee to foods is prominent in our culture, but the ghee that we used to get years ago is difficult to find now. Ghee made at home should be made from organic milk from cows that have been left in the pastures to graze and not given hormones to increase milk production. The reliability of commercial organic products is suspect, so make sure you do your homework on the organic product, so you are not wasting your money and eating unhealthily.

So, what do you do about weight gain during cancer treatment? Do not go on a diet to lose weight during your treatment. Talk to your doctor, find out why you are gaining weight, and discuss what course of action to take. You may think of cutting unhealthy calories if it is your food intake. But if you are gaining weight or have gained weight from your cancer treatments, just be aware of it, as keeping a healthy weight is a very valuable tool for a positive outcome. Research conducted over the last few years has established the importance of maintaining a healthy weight and staying as lean as possible without being underweight for cancer survivors. Having a healthy weight seems to establish a biochemical status or "anti-cancer" environment that discourages cancer growth. The research shows that carrying extra body fat, particularly excess abdominal fat, puts you at higher risk for certain cancers. Homemade real foods, an active lifestyle, and daily yogic practices can help with natural healthy weight loss.

Sweet Cravings

We advocate eating no sugar or as little sugar as possible during treatment, but after treatment ends and you want to feel as normal as possible, perhaps start eating the foods you once did. If you are missing your sweet dishes, you can begin to introduce healthy desserts to your diet, in moderation, of course. Desserts sweetened with jaggery, honey, and liquid jaggery can be introduced. Just remember that sweets are calorific even if they are seemingly healthy. Recipes for a few healthy desserts are mentioned in the Appendix.

Weight Loss, Cachexia, and Anorexia

Unintentional weight loss is not uncommon during treatment. Maintaining your weight can be challenging, especially if you are experiencing side effects of treatment. Loss of appetite leads to malnutrition, weight loss, and decreased immunity to infections. However, anorexia during cancer is different from the widely known eating disorder Anorexia Nervosa.

Anorexia during cancer treatment is caused by a number of factors, including the side effects of treatment such as nausea, vomiting, and mouth sores, all of which lower the desire to eat. Many tumors produce chemicals that disrupt the endocrine system, which provides the sensation of satiety (feeling full) faster. Gastrointestinal surgeries or tumors can also lower the desire to eat. Here are a few solutions:

- Appetite is usually the best first thing in the morning, so plan to have a large meal for breakfast.
- Eat many small meals or snacks instead of 3 big ones, or eat bites of nutrient-dense foods every hour or so.
- Eat whenever you feel hungry. Do not wait for regular mealtimes.
- Try not to smell food. If possible, steer clear of the kitchen, or keep food odors to a minimum.
- Liquids are often more appealing than solid foods when you are

Our patient, Mrs. Oswal developed a bad case of dyspepsia during her third round of chemo. She had little discomfort during her first two rounds, but this round was taking its toll and she started rejecting her favorite foods. The mere sight and smell of the food was making her sick, and she began losing weight. We suggested these measures for Mrs. Oswal to help mitigate her weight loss.

- *She was asked not to look at the food while eating.*
- *The TV was shifted to her terrace, far from the kitchen, and she was advised to watch comedy shows and movies while eating.*
- *Her caretaker was told to serve cold food so that the aroma would not offend her.*
- *Before eating, she was advised to chew on a piece of garlic dipped in salt.*
- *We prescribed a sound mixture.*

experiencing side effects of treatment. Fresh vegetable and fruit juices can replace whole vegetables and fruits. Watered-down dals and curries can be eaten as soups. Tomato *saar*, *sol kadhi*, and lemon coriander soup are examples of foods packed with needed vitamins and minerals. See a few recipes and ideas in Appendix II.

- Do not drink water with meals. You will feel full faster.
- Eat the most nutrient-dense foods on the *thali* first. For example, start the meal with 2-3 spoons of *sabzi* and dals.
- Avoid low-calorie, low-protein foods and beverages such as tea, coffee, and sodas. These beverages and water as well, will kill

your appetite and fill you up with lesser amounts of protein and calories.

- Avoid raw vegetables. The high fiber content may not be good for your system when experiencing extreme weight loss. Steam or cook vegetables with high-density foods such as nuts and seeds.
- Light exercise may improve your appetite. Ask your doctor if you can take a short walk before mealtimes.
- Mealtimes should be relaxed and appealing. Use nice plates and *katoris*, tablecloths – anything that makes you happy.
- Very sour foods such as *amla*, raw mango, or tamarind candy may stimulate the appetite. One lemon mixed with a teaspoon of sugar is also an option. A taste of these mixtures throughout the day will help activate the taste buds.
- Add homemade protein powder to foods (see recipe for homemade protein powder in Appendix II).
- Eat nutrient-dense foods such as:
  - *Parathas* (*aloo*/pumpkin)
  - *Palak puri*
  - Stuffed vegetables
  - Dal cutlet
  - Egg/paneer *bhurji*
  - Indian pancakes (*cheela*, *dosa*, etc.)
  - Dry fruits
  - Smoothies
- Radiation may affect taste buds, making food taste bitter or metallic. Using non-metal vessels and utensils may help; use melamine plates and bamboo spoons instead of the standard steel. Also, our Indian tradition of eating with our hands is useful in this situation.

Post-Cancer Exercise

Cachexia and sarcopenia are two conditions that can happen post radiotherapy or post chemotherapy. Cancer cachexia is the wasting of muscles while sarcopenia is the loss of muscle mass due lack of use. Even after successfully being in remission, some cancer patients still experience both side-effects. The conditions are more prevalent with those with advanced cancers.

During and after cancer, most patients are not able to move around and do their daily chores as they once did. Exercise should be an important part of cancer treatment but unfortunately this is not the case. In our practices, we have found that relatives of cancer patients do not allow patients to do their routine housework, let alone exercise. Cancer fatigue is real, and it is normal for the cancer patient to need to sleep for hours. But unfortunately, sarcopenia develops quickly and can lead to a reduced quality of life post cancer therapy.

Cancer cachexia causes reduction in strength and stamina and sometimes one has trouble getting up from the floor without taking external support. This weakness cycles into more weakness as the patient is not motivated to move around, all of which takes a toll on their overall health, putting additional strain on the caregivers as well. Psychological counseling is helpful at this stage as the patient should understand that the worst part of cancer treatment is over, and life can begin to be normal again.

An important thing to note here is that sarcopenia will not improve through quality diet or medication, but only through weight bearing exercises. It is important to identify this muscle loss at an early stage and treat it before it is too late.

Oncologists ask caregivers to keep an eye on the weight of the patient and a weight loss of more than 5% needs attention. Patients and their caregivers need to be vigilant about symptoms such as weight loss, loss of appetite, weakness, and mental distress and inform their doctor. Cachexia is usually treated with high carbohydrate protein powders along with higher calorie diet plans.

Post-cancer sarcopenia can be prevented with the practice of weight bearing exercises, which can significantly reduce incidences of post-cancer muscle and joint disorders. Initially, this is best done under the supervision of a physiotherapist. Fatigue, which is a common symptom for cancer patients, is a major hurdle in making the patient exercise regularly during and after treatment. But those patients who do some regular physical activity benefit not just physically but mentally as well. Exercise is a natural anti-depressant, stress buster.

Post recovery, cancer survivors are also at risk of certain lifestyle diseases such as type-2 diabetes and cardiovascular disease, making it even more important to invest the time and effort into physical activity once conventional cancer treatment is over.

To look out for sarcopenia after treatment check for the following:

- You are unable to get up from the floor without taking support of both your hands.
- You start getting muscle pain and stiffness in the winter season.
- You start experiencing backache after sitting for a long time.

- Your handshake becomes less robust due to a weakening grip strength.
- You feel that your stamina is gradually reducing.

Resistance exercise is the best line of treatment for sarcopenia – easy to perform, cost effective, and gives results. Having a physiotherapist guide you a few times will ensure you are doing the exercises correctly.

Hip abduction, straight leg raises, knee extensions, hip extensions, and calf raises are a few examples of exercises you should include for muscle strengthening. The amount of resistance, repetitions, duration, etc. will be suggested by your physiotherapist and will increase over time.

Yoga Post-Cancer

In Chapter 6, (Movement is Medicine) we have written in detail about the benefits of yoga. The importance of this 3000-year-old tradition cannot be emphasized enough. The true aim of yoga is to attain self-realization and one of the first steps towards achieving this is to prepare the body with different *asanas*. *Asanas* develop strength, stability, stamina, concentration, and body alignment – all in a safe and gentle manner, which is crucial post-chemo and post-radiation.

Right after cancer treatment protocol is finished, it may not be possible to do many active poses. Chemo and radiation weaken the body and it is important to be gentle with the body during treatment and post treatment. One can begin with sitting and supine *asanas*. Incorporating regular pranayama and meditation will help you alleviate stress and increase your lung capacity.

Resistance against the pull of gravity puts stress on our bones. *Asanas* that involve weight bearing on the bones such as standing and balancing *asanas* increase the active resistance of our bones against gravity, improving bone health. When you are able to do standing *asanas* you will get the benefit of muscle strengthening.

Author's Closing Notes

Dr. Seema Sonis

Everyone knows someone whom the disease of cancer has touched. I have had several relatives who have had cancer – colon, laryngeal, breast, and cervical. All are living healthy lives today. There are two women who I love and respect and whose stories I would like to share. Both women, thriving today, used holistic techniques to help the healing process but approached their disease differently.

Thirty years ago, my mother was diagnosed with endometrial cancer when she was in her 40s and at the peak of her career. Cancer was much more frightening back then, and survival rates were lower. An Ayurvedic doctor herself, she decided to tackle the endometrial cancer head-on. She was angry she got sick and literally went to war with her cancer. A workaholic without the best lifestyle practices, she knew she needed help. After her Surgery and on the way to recovery, she made the decision, much to my disapproval, to check into a holistic treatment center. She completely shut off from the world – she gave up meat, ate wholesome vegetarian meals, and practiced yoga and meditation every day – all things she knew were good for her but never applied. I remember visiting her and seeing her plate full of colorful fruits and vegetables, not a usual sight on my mother's plate. I had just begun my practice and did not understand the power of yoga and healing foods at the time, but I am happy to report that my Mom is full of life today, even at the age of 75, she has more energy than me!

My sister-in-law, Jyostna, was the epitome of health, shocking everyone with her breast cancer diagnosis. How could such a fit person eating well and living right get cancer? When I heard the news, I rushed to visit her and was surprised at how rational and calm she was. She accepted her diagnosis with an unattached calmness, in an almost Zen-type way. She was not angry but curious. She began to read about malignancy and was proactive in her healing, asking the oncologists about treatment options. She discussed nutritional support with me and went to a holistic practitioner for supplemental support. She gave up meat and white sugar and increased the number of fruits, salads, and cooked vegetables in her diet. Dairy products, bakery foods, and wheat were minimized. Jyostna appreciated the love and support of her family; she embraced the calmness and took to meditating and practicing gratitude. She overcame the strong chemotherapy and radiation sessions and today, she is stronger than before.

My co-author Rita and I have written this book for many reasons. After seeing so many patients in our practice who do not know how to alleviate their side effects due to chemo and radiation, we knew there was a need for this information to be easily available. Very few books, if any, have a rational narrative with an Indian perspective on dealing with cancer. India has the right tools to fight cancer. We have the privilege of the latest modern medicine and the traditional wisdom of Ayurveda and yogic sciences. More importantly, India has a rich collection of fruits, vegetables, grains, herbs, and spices. Potent tools of healing are present right in our kitchen. And ingrained in our culture are yoga and Ayurveda, as is religion. The philosophical teaching of the Bhagavad Gita or any religious texts of other faiths can give us the resilience of mind. Through *Fighting Cancer with the Thali*, we want to convey that one can overcome cancer using conventional modern medicine combined with our traditional Indian healing modalities.

FAQs

Following is a compilation of the most frequently asked questions by our cancer patients and caregivers.

Should I take nutritional supplements for cancer prevention? During treatment? After treatment?

Thousands of studies over the years have uncovered a clear and distinct relationship between vital nutrients and cancer risk. However, there is no reliable evidence that any nutritional supplement can help prevent cancer. However, there is evidence that a healthy diet incorporating plenty of fruits and vegetables can reduce your cancer risk.

A balanced diet with the right nutrients is the only way to reduce your risk. Cancer is caused by uncontrolled cell proliferation. How this happens is yet unknown, but we know that many carcinogens damage our DNA, and when DNA becomes damaged, genes start to mutate or change form. Our cells need to protect their DNA. To do this, cells need the right nutrients at the right times.

India's population is deficient in certain nutrients, such as Vitamin D and B12. Nearly 50% of Indian women are deficient in iron. In these cases, supplementation is necessary to live a healthy life and prevent diseases such as cancer. When undergoing treatment, however, you should ask your doctor about supplementation. Certain supplements may interfere with chemotherapy drugs as well as radiation therapy.

Also, never assume something herbal or natural is safe. For example, adding some ginger to your food or tea is healthy, but producers of supplements with ginger in it claim it curbs nausea, a treatment side-effect. High doses of this spice concentrated into a pill are not so safe, especially when you are undergoing treatment. Different medications have different reactions to active compounds of the spices, so it is best to ask your oncologist if supplements are needed.

Post-treatment, again, it is recommended to ask your doctor which supplements are best suited for your medical condition. Herbal supplements may not be as harmful at this point but use caution when choosing what to put in your body. Many supplements cause constipation too. Good digestion is vital to health, and having trouble with bowel movements can hinder your return to a normal state of health. The supplement market is a big business that growing due to the health claims they make. You may be wasting thousands of rupees on unnecessary pills.

In short, if you want to try herbal remedies, it's best to take them in their natural state after asking your doctor. For instance, instead of taking green tea capsules, drink a cup of green tea. Unless you have a specific, targeted reason to take curcumin tablets, which contain the compound found in turmeric, there is no need, as this spice is amply included in our diet.

I am vegetarian. What foods can I eat to increase my iron levels?

If you wish to enhance your hemoglobin naturally, here is a list of vegetarian sources of high-iron foods:
- Green leafy vegetables
- Beans such as soybeans and kidney beans

- Whole grains – bajra and wheat
- Dry fruits – black currants, raisins, dates, apricots
- Oil seeds – sesame, Niger seeds
- Green chutneys – mint, coriander
- Spices – fenugreek, cumin, coriander seeds, turmeric, *ajwain*
- Herbs – holy basil (*tulsi*), wheatgrass
- Fruits – watermelon
- Other – dark chocolate
- Use iron vessels for cooking

To enhance iron absorption in the intestine, have one *amla* or one lemon or 1-2 oranges daily. Limit the consumption of tea, coffee, and aerated drinks.

How do I calculate BMI?

The formula for BMI is: kg/m^2 where Kg is your weight and m^2 is your height in meters squared. A BMI of 25.0 or more is overweight, while the healthy range is 18.5 to 24.9. 25-30 is considered acceptable. 30-35 is obese and above 35 is morbidly obese. BMI applies to most adults 18-65 years.

Can I have milk?

There is no strict rule against milk, but many patients cannot tolerate drinking plain milk during treatment. If this is the case, please do not drink it. There are plenty of other sources of calcium, such as yogurt, green leafy vegetables, seeds, and nuts. Drinking milk has been a historic part of our food culture; drinking it at night is believed to be healthy, promoting sound sleep. The age-old turmeric milk remedy helps alleviate sore throats and colds.

The fact is that healthy dairy products are not readily available in India and the ones offered are prohibitively expensive for most of the population. Studies over the past few decades have pointed clearly to the fact that the meat or byproducts of cattle fed artificial growth hormones have increased breast cancer, obesity, and early puberty in the United States. Large-scale dairy production in India also incorporates these hormones so it can be assumed that we are also at risk of these conditions if we consume a substantial amount of dairy.

We suggest *dahi* as the better option since it offers some good bacteria. Both curds and buttermilk should be staples in the *thali*. Many of our patients find that they can tolerate *dahi* and buttermilk but can no longer drink milk.

What is Gir cow's milk?

Desi Cow's Milk, also known as Gir's milk or A2 milk, has gained popularity as the healthier milk. Currently, the evidence does support this. The desi breed of cows has a unique hump on their back, and studies have shown that sun rays enter the cow's body through the hump, making their milk, dung, and urine medicinal (Hajare, 2017).

The main difference between crossbred cow's milk and desi cow's milk is that the former contains A1 protein and the latter A2 protein. A2 type of protein is found to be easily digestible, high in omega-3, and richer in antioxidants and related nutrients. Desi-bred cow's milk is believed to offer protection from ailments like gout, asthma, obesity, heart disease, migraine headaches, and arthritis, among others. It also protects colon cells from chemicals that cause cancer.

A 2012 report published in the Indian journal of Endocrinology and Metabolism states that the A1 protein is associated with an increased risk of coronary heart disease and mental disorders like autism and schizophrenia. So why did India start using crossbreed cow's milk in the first place? In 1970 there was a milk scarcity in the country and to correct it, the Indian government launched a program called operation flood, which transformed India into one of the largest milk-producing nations in the world. But sadly, this 'white revolution' led to cross breeding with foreign cows for higher yields in order to meet the nation's goal of mass production.

Today, the benefits of desi cow's milk and milk products is spreading and leading to conservation activities for native breeds in certain regions of India. As the Indian breed gives only 8 liters of milk while the cross-breeds produce 15-20 liters, the former type is considerably more expensive. But keep in mind that disease management is expensive too! Common desi breeds are *geer, sahiwal, red sindhi, rathi,* and *tharparkar. Veeshur,* one of Kerala's healthiest breeds of desi cows, is sadly on the brink of extinction.

Should I avoid sugar?

During cancer treatment, you should try and give up white sugar. Let's understand in simpler terms what happens when we eat highly refined food products like sugar and white flour. Foods made with these ingredients have a very high glycemic index (GI). Glycemic index is an indicator of how quickly the food causes a rise in blood glucose levels when eaten. When we eat foods with high GI, the body immediately releases a dose of insulin to enable glucose to enter the cells. The secretion of insulin is accompanied by a molecule called insulin-like growth factor (IGF). IGF stimulates cell growth. All our cells need glucose for nourishment. But this supply of glucose has to arrive in a controlled way. High GI foods like sugar boost blood glucose levels, thus resulting in equally high levels of insulin and IGF. Such a biochemical condition is not considered healthy. In the malignant state, fast-growing cancer cells are nourished by this high supply of glucose. In other words, more glucose, more cell growth. In 1931, German biologist Otto Warburg won the Nobel prize in medicine for his discovery that the metabolism of malignant tumors largely depends on glucose consumption. Today, we know that peaks of insulin and IGF directly stimulate the growth of cancer cells and their ability to spread to other parts of the body.

After treatment, patients want to feel normal and eat normally. It is natural that rigid restrictions like eating absolutely no sugar will wane. Eating a bit of unrefined sugar is okay at this point. Some healthy dessert recipes are included in Appendix II.

Should I Avoid Soy?

Soy is not a staple on our *thali*, nevertheless, it is a myth that it contributes to cancer. Soy is a plant food, usually consumed in whole food forms like edamame, tofu, soy nuts, and soy milk, providing a good source of protein. Eating whole plant foods like these is better for you than the concentrated soy found in supplements and processed foods made with soy protein isolates. Like all plant foods, soy contains phytonutrients/phytochemicals, which make plant foods good for you. Regarding soy foods in relation to breast or endometrial type cancers, soy contains some phytoestrogens that are plant estrogens. This phytochemical in soy appears similar to the human estrogen in chemical structure, but soy plants do not grow human estrogen; they are only chemically similar. Commercial soya chunks available in the market are okay to have.

Can I Have Alcohol?

Alcohol has been proven to raise the risk of cancer.

There are conflicting studies on whether red wine helps with cancer protection, but we do not consider wine drinking an essential part of an anti-cancer healthy diet. Red wine has been touted as a heart-healthy alcohol because it contains the compound resveratrol. Resveratrol is also found in other plant foods such as peanuts, red grapes, blueberries, and dark chocolate. Peanuts and grapes are available all over India, and peanuts are widely used in our *thalis*. In the Mediterranean diet, which is supposed to be one of the healthiest diets in the world, wine drinking is moderate and incorporated with food. Indian wine connoisseurs may try and sell the idea that wine goes well with Indian food. But that is just not the case.

If you enjoy drinking, then drink moderately. Moderate alcohol consumption is defined as having up to 1 drink per day for women and up to 2 drinks per day for men. This is the amount you drink in one day and not the average over several days. And if you do not drink, please do not start, even if studies indicate that red wine is good for your heart. When patients ask us if they should drink wine for their heart, we respond by asking them if they are doing everything else necessary for a healthy heart. Is the rest of your nutrition optimal? Are you getting regular physical activity, and what method are you using to handle any stress you may have?

What is an Alkaline Diet? Do I need to have an Alkaline Diet?

It makes sense to eat a majority of alkaline foods: fruits and vegetables. This is exactly what we are recommending, that 50% of the *thali* should contain both cooked and raw vegetables.

The internet is filled with websites claiming alkaline diets not only ward off disease but actually help cure it, including cancer. However, there is no scientific basis for this claim. The myth is that cancer thrives in an acidic environment, and by eating alkaline foods, you can starve cancer cells. Our body's pH level is well-regulated and remains around 7.4 on a scale of 1-14.

Although no research indicates that the alkaline diet wards off disease, the diet's premise makes it healthy. In short, fruits and vegetables are alkaline, animal foods, including dairy, are acidic, and whole grains and pulses fall somewhere in between. During treatment, however, protein needs are high, and an alkaline diet does not advocate eating any animal protein, so ensure you get enough of it through other sources. Our traditional vegetarian *thali* is alkaline, minus the fried items, *dahi* and sweets. However, dairy in the form of *dahi* and cheese are good sources of protein, calcium, and probiotics.

Alkaline water is marketed as being helpful with your pH levels, something that actually cannot be changed by drinking or eating. Drinking it will not harm you, but it is just a waste of money.

Here is a list of some Alkaline Foods:
- Cereals – Rice, Ragi, Rajgeera, Jowar
- Dals – Green gram, Red lentil, Sprouts (cooked), Pulses
- Sweet Potato, Potato, *Shingada*
- Jaggery (chemical free)
- Raisins
- Non-veg foods with green salad and lemon/pomegranate
- Cold milk, Fresh yogurt, Fresh buttermilk, Pure ghee
- Guava, Banana, Chickoo, Custard Apple, Mango, *Jambhul*, Blackberry (*karvanda*), Muskmelon, Watermelon, Pomegranate, Lemon, *Amla*
- All Gourds, all root vegetables, all green leafy vegetables
- Herbs like coriander and mint
- Masalas/Spices – Coriander seeds, Cumin seeds, Cardamom
- Traditional homemade balanced meals

Here is a list of some Acidic Foods:
- Cereals – Wheat, Corn, Bajra
- Dals – *Toor* dal, All unsprouted pulses, Soyabean
- *Sago*, *Varai*, Groundnut
- White Sugar
- Sugarcane juice
- Liquid jaggery (*kakwi*)
- All types of non-veg foods
- Sour Curds, Paneer, Cheese
- Raw mango, Unripe citrus fruits, Tamarind

- Mustard, Pepper, Chili
- All types of Junk foods
- Canned foods

What are some vegetarian sources of protein?

Nutrients such as Vitamin B, iron, and protein are more difficult to acquire from plant sources alone, but not impossible. Unless you are an athlete, your body needs 0.8 grams of protein per kilo of body weight. A person weighing 60 kgs needs 48 grams of protein. One *katori* of dal, one *katori* of pulses, and one *katori* of *dahi* contain about 18 grams of protein. Protein is found in nearly all foods that we eat: nuts, seeds, and grains, which are also part of the *thali*. Paneer has protein, but portions need to be limited as it is high in fat. All our pulses have higher amounts of proteins, as do traditional grains such as *rajgira*, ragi, and *bajra*. Soya in the form of tofu and soya chunks is also a good option. A large number of our population is non-vegetarian however in India many non-vegetarians do not eat meat on a daily basis, so it is important for them to keep an eye on their protein intake.

What are some vegetarian sources of iron? Do I need supplements?

Nearly 50% of Indian women are iron-deficient. Unfortunately, iron is difficult to acquire from food, at least at needed levels, and supplementation is necessary if your hemoglobin levels are low.

Can I have coffee?

For decades, there has been ongoing research on the effects of coffee on cancer. As of now, there is no conclusive evidence that coffee causes cancer or affects any treatment protocol. If you enjoy coffee, have it in moderation.

Should I take wheatgrass juice? Does it cure cancer?

It does not cure cancer in any way. It is a healthy drink with plenty of fiber, vitamins, and minerals; you can include it in a healthy diet. If you are undergoing cancer treatment, you must be mindful if it interacts with your digestion or has side effects.

Where do I get blueberries?

You do not have to eat blueberries! They are one of the "superfoods" you read about but are not widely cultivated in India, if at all. If you find them after spending loads of money, remember that they have traveled a long distance and have probably been preserved to withstand the journey. There are in fact, plenty of Indian berries that can also be considered superfoods. Gooseberries, mulberries, Indian blueberries (*jambhul*) and Indian blackberries (*kharvanda*) are also high in the ORAC value.

Which oil should I use?

Refined oils are the most commonly used oils in Indian homes because they are economical and easily available. Unfortunately, they are the worst oils for your health. Refined oils are extracted using chemical solvents at very high temperatures, which leads to the formation of trans fats. After this, a neutralization process is performed by adding preservatives and anti-foaming agents. This results in a colorless, flavorless, odorless oil completely devoid of all nutritive components of the original oil seed.

Extra virgin olive oil is a healthy option but is not affordable for a majority of the population. The composition of olive oil makes it unsuitable for the high smoke points our Indian cooking requires, though extra-virgin olive oil is good for salads or light stir fries.

Pomace olive oil is marketed in stores as a healthy oil with a high smoke point, making it more adaptable to Indian cooking, but it is also highly processed and as unhealthy as any other refined oil.

The best oils to use in India are readily available cold-pressed (*kachchi-ghani*) oils such as sesame, coconut, groundnut, and mustard. Since no high heat is involved in the extraction process, the natural properties of the oils are preserved. These oils have a high smoking point and are suitable to the Indian way of cooking. Pure ghee made at home is also a good cooking medium. Ghee does not burn easily, as it has a high smoking point, and does not generate free radicals when heated.

How much oil should one have?

600ml per month, per person or 20ml per adult per day is the recommended amount of visible fats.

How much ghee is good?

Pure ghee or clarified butter is an essential part of Indian meals. Since ghee is non-refined and devoid of chemicals, it can be safely incorporated into your daily meals if it comes from a good source. The beta-carotene in cow's ghee is an antioxidant, which is cancer-protective. We suggest using ghee as the cooking medium in one of the three main daily meals. Mr. Amit Vaidya, who fought cancer by radically changing his lifestyle and eating habits, advocates the use of cow's ghee by cancer patients. In his book 'Holy Cancer: How a cow saved my life' Mr. Vaidya describes daily yoga practices, 10 km walks, opting for organic foods and herbs like tulsi and neem, and the daily use of cow's milk and ghee. Please keep in mind that ghee is saturated animal fat and should be used in moderate amounts. If you wish to take pure ghee as a topping on your rice or parathas, then 1-2 teaspoons (5-10ml) a day is what we advise.

Can I exercise during treatment?

Yes! The benefits of physical activity are enormous. Even moderate exercise lifts your mood, assists cardiovascular function, and helps you overcome fatigue. Before beginning any exercise routine, get an okay from your doctor (see Chapter 13 for more on cancer and yoga).

Can I have ice cream?

If you are craving something during treatment, then go ahead. Just ensure you do not overindulge so that you leave room for healthy calories as well.

Should I drink green tea?

If you like it, drink it. Black tea is just as good.

Can I eat at restaurants?

Whether it is for the ambiance, social connection, or just some food you would like to eat, there will be times you'll feel like eating out. Just stick to the 80-20 rule in which 80% of your meals are healthy and home-cooked. If you are having trouble eating due to a sore mouth or nausea, eating at restaurants may help you get some calories you're lacking. You'll have more food choices in restaurants and will generally be kept away from strong food smells. Here are a few eating out tips:

- Go early to avoid crowds. Wait staff will be more accommodating if there are fewer guests.
- Go to reputable restaurants where hygiene is paramount. This may be more expensive, but it is not negotiable. In any case, you will be going out less frequently, so it is okay to spend that money.
- Order multiple side dishes rather than one main dish. You can taste more foods and eat the ones you like.
- Select dishes from the children's menu. You will get smaller portions there.
- Continue to avoid raw foods such as salads and chutneys.
- Drink bottled water.

Should I eat an anti-angiogenic diet?

Angiogenesis is the process your body uses to build blood vessels. When tumors grow, they often build blood vessels that connect to the body's circulatory system. These vessels provide the pathways for nutrients that tumors need to continue their expansion, making the tumor or disease worse. Research suggests that compounds found in certain foods, such as green tea, red grapes, turmeric, and strawberries, may also inhibit angiogenesis. Almost all anti-angiogenic foods are fruits or vegetables – no big surprise. A balanced diet would include foods that are not on the list of anti-angiogenic foods, such as whole grains, pulses, nuts, and lean protein like fish. We advise balancing all elements of food.

Do you have any suggestions for caregivers who are too tired to cook?

A few shortcuts for cooking are:

- When the patient needs to be on a liquid diet, use nutritional meal supplements so they can get all the needed nutrients. Making and blending food can be time-consuming and exhausting when you have to do it for 3 meals a day, every day.
- For a more cost-effective alternative to meal replacement, you can add protein powder to baby cereal such as Cerelac. This is a complete meal and gives a nutritional boost to a patient who cannot eat the whole foods needed.
- If you are cooking, make large batches of food and freeze half. You can use frozen foods when you are too busy or tired to cook.
- Patients are often hungriest at the start of the day. If that is the case, prepare the largest meal in the morning.
- Keep healthy chutneys on hand (see more on chutneys in Chapter 3).
- Don't stress about perfectly balanced meals. There will be some good days and bad days.

- Try new foods. Tastes change during treatment, and something new may be more palatable to the patient than what they have been eating before.

Should I drink juice?

If the juice is made fresh at home, you can drink it. Vegetables and fruits are what we promote, so if juicing is the way you want to have them, then go ahead. However, think about blending instead. Smoothies, which are blended, retain fiber, whereas juicing requires that you strain out the fiber to create a clear liquid.

Do I need to eat organic foods?

Pesticides and chemicals are pervasive in food today – the toxins present in these foods are feared to be carcinogenic. If you have an option of eating organic foods, then you should opt for them. Many companies are touting the organic label, and it may be difficult to know if they are genuine. Our advice is to have faith and trust, and don't stress thinking whether you are being cheated. Groceries have to be purchased, and if there is a choice, then have confidence and buy the organic label.

Are charred meats bad for you?

Cooking meat at very high temperatures (grilling, broiling, tandoor) causes the amino acids in fish, chicken, beef, and pork to form chemicals called heterocyclic amines (HCA's). Also carcinogenic chemicals are formed as the fat drips into the hot grill coals and is redeposited back onto the meat by smoke. These chemicals have been found to increase the risk of developing cancer. Avoid having tandoor or grilled non-veg on a regular basis. Curry-based, slow cooked non-veg or shallow fried in pan on medium heat is a better option.

Can I try Ayurvedic or Homeopathic medications?

In India, we have no dearth of non-allopathic treatments. For ages, Ayurveda has complemented our traditional way of living. Yoga, meditation, and pranayama originated here. Homeopathy and naturopathy have been prevalent in India for over a century before they became popular in the West.

When you get a cancer diagnosis, you feel out of control but want to try anything that may save your life. Alternative treatments make you feel as though you have some of that control. Perhaps your friends or family members advise you to try other treatments before taking harmful chemo and radiation, or you read online about all sorts of natural cures for cancer. At the moment, only mainstream oncology treatment has been proven to cure cancer.

People with cancer who choose alternative medicine are giving up the mainstream approach to treating their disease. If you delay or interrupt your standard cancer treatment in any way, it can give cancer more time to grow.

If there have been people who have been cured of their cancer naturally, they are not the norm, as this happens in extremely rare cases. Also, no conclusive clinical trials have been performed on humans that prove any alternative treatments work. This type of research is needed to prove treatments are successful. Many new allopathic drugs found to be useful in treating lab animals were shown to not work in humans. So, they were never brought to use. Extensive clinical trials, including tests on humans in a clinical setting, are completed on allopathic cancer drugs before they are considered effective. The results of such studies are published in credible peer-reviewed journals studied by scientists and doctors in the field.

It's important to understand the distinction between 'alternative' and 'complementary'. Alternative medicine is used instead of allopathy, whereas 'complementary' is as it sounds – it complements allopathy.

Presently, alternative medicine can be used to complement cancer treatment, especially to alleviate side effects. Many foods and principles in Ayurveda and naturopathy are excellent for supporting resilience and combating certain side effects such as nausea, dry mouth, and other related symptoms.

Ask your oncologist if you are thinking of taking any non-allopathic medication (including supplements and herbs) during your cancer treatment, as there are substances that can interfere with chemo drugs.

How often should I get preventive health checks?

As a well-being measure, preventive health checkups are necessary. We recommend preventive nutritional tests for everyone, as deficiencies can lead to many health problems. We often find that cancer patients have underlying nutrient deficiencies when they get blood tests during treatment. Specifically, Hemoglobin, Vitamin B12, and Vitamin D3 should be checked annually. These preventive nutritional tests will help you detect any deficiencies at the right time.

These deficiencies are affordable and easy to treat. More importantly, a nutritionally balanced body can fight off cancer more effectively. In India, iron deficiency, also known as anemia, is common, especially in women who have been untreated for the condition for a long time. Anemia leads to low immunity status and chronic fatigue. A simple yearly Hemoglobin test followed by doctor-prescribed supplementation can be useful as cancer treatment often causes the red blood cell count to drop further, worsening the anemia.

Vitamin B12 is a heart-protective and energy-producing vitamin. B12 deficiency is quite common in India since its dietary sources are not a regular part of the Indian diet. Though Vitamin B12 has no direct connection with the prevention or treatment of cancer, it is a vitamin that protects us from physical and mental fatigue. Fatigue is one of the most common side effects of cancer treatment and often the most difficult to treat. We have observed that detecting B12 deficiency and treating it promptly with supplements has helped a considerable number of cancer patients post-treatment. People suffering from low energy levels, vague muscular pains, tingling in the feet, forgetfulness, and mood swings can benefit immensely from B12 supplementation.

Vitamin D3 is an important fat-soluble vitamin present only in animal foods. Most people know that Vitamin D is needed for calcium absorption, but it plays a much bigger role in the body. Vitamin D protects from 3 major ailments:

- Diabetes
- Depression
- Cancer

Vitamin D deficiency cannot be diagnosed clinically. One can be severely Vitamin D deficient and still have no complaints or telltale signs. Only a blood test can diagnose this condition. Though the test is currently expensive, the treatment for Vitamin D deficiency is quite cheap and simple. We recommend annual check-ups of Vitamin D3, especially if you have a history of cancer or diabetes in the family. Others may check it every two years.

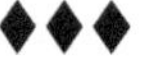

Probiotics

Homemade Dahi (Yogurt)

Ingredients
- 1 liter of milk
- 2 tbsp of *dahi* as a starter (purchase dahi from a local dairy)

Directions
1. Boil the milk and let it cool. Put a finger in it. The mixture should be warm, but if you feel like taking out your finger because it is too warm, let it cool for a few more minutes. Add the starter and stir to spread evenly. Set in a corner overnight and refrigerate when set, usually 8-10 hours.
2. If your doctor has told you to avoid dairy or if you just feel that you want to avoid it but still want to eat your curds, try making curds with soy milk or nut milk, made at home or bought from a good source.

Soy Curds

(for those who want to avoid dairy)

Ingredients

- 75 gms Soybeans
- 1.5 liters of water

Directions

1. For Soy Milk: Soak the 75 grams of soybeans in water for 24 hours, then ground to a fine paste. Add one liter of water and grind again and stir until even. Sieve through a cheese-cloth or a fine sieve to make the milk.
2. For Curds: Boil the soy milk and proceed to make curds using the directions for the homemade *dahi* recipe above. You will need some soy curds to use as a starter.

Note: You can also make curds with almond and oat milk.

Pazhaya Saadam (fermented rice)

This procedure creates a natural fermentation process. Rice, a resilient starch, acts as a nutritious feed for the good bacteria in our colon. It also heals the gut lining, thus increasing the functional capacity of the intestine. The botanic acid in the fermented rice reduces the inflammation of the colon.

Ingredients

- Leftover Rice
- Water
- Curds (optional)
- Green chilies, curry leaves (optional)
- Salt to taste

Directions

1. Place leftover rice in a clay pot and cover it with water about one inch above the rice. Leave overnight. Have 1-2 tablespoons in the morning.
2. Optionally, you can add curds and some flavor, such as green chilies, curry leaves, and salt.

Kanji Vada (Fried mung balls from Rajasthan)

Ingredients

- 8 cups of water
- 4 tsp of salt
- 9 tsp of mustard dal

For Vada -

- 1 cup of green *moong* dal
- 1 tsp of red chili powder
- 1 tsp of coriander powder
- 1 tbsp of coriander (fresh)
- 1 tsp of finely chopped ginger
- pinch soda bicarb
- oil for frying

Directions

1. In an earthen pot, mix water, salt, red chili, and mustard dal.
2. Soak *moong* dal for 4 hours and then grind to a paste.
3. Add the coriander powder, fresh coriander, ginger, and soda bicarb to the dal paste and mix well.
4. Form small round balls and fry till golden brown. Let cool.
5. Put these *vadas* into the earthen pot water and keep them in a warm place for 2-3 days.

Snacks

Drumstick Flower Cutlets

Ingredients

- 1 cup drumstick flowers
- 1 cup shredded coconut (fresh/frozen)
- ½ cup toor dal
- 2 tsp rice flour
- 2 tsp *besan* flour
- 1 tsp coriander seeds
- 2 tsp *urad* dal
- ¼ tsp asafoetida
- ½ tsp tamarind extract
- 4-5 red chillies
- 2 tsp jaggery
- Salt
- Oil
- *Rava*

Directions

1. Soak tur dal in water for about thirty minutes.
2. Heat a little oil and fry coriander seeds, *urad* dal, asafoetida and red chillies.
3. Grind coconut, jaggery, rice flour, tamarind and above fried items. Continue grinding with soaked dal and salt using minimum water. Mix this masala with drumstick flowers.
4. Make small balls, roll them in *rava* and flatten on the *tava* to shallow fry them with a bit of oil. Fry on both sides.

Healthy Desserts

Banana Appe

This is a good alternative to bakery products. Ragi, rice, and carrots are alkaline foods, and coconut has healthy fats. Bananas are prebiotic.

Ingredients

- ½ cup of ragi flour
- ½ cup of rice flour
- ½ cup of grated carrots
- ½ cup of grated fresh coconut
- ½ cup of smashed banana
- ½ cup of organic jaggery
- Pinch of salt
- 1 tsp of baking soda
- Ghee for greasing the pan

Directions

1. Melt and dilute the jaggery in some boiling hot water to make thin jaggery syrup.
2. Mix all the ingredients and the jaggery liquid. Let the mixture sit for 30 minutes.
3. Apply ghee to the *appe* pan. Put batter in pan and roast on both sides until golden brown (about 10 minutes).

Carrot Laddoos

Carrots and sesame are good sources of antioxidants, and this is a delicious alternative to calorie-laden *mithais*.

Ingredients

- ½ cup of grated carrots
- ¼ cup of powdered jaggery
- ¼ cup of grated fresh coconut
- ¼ cup of milk powder
- 1 tbsp of milk
- A handful of sesame seeds

Directions

1. Add carrots, jaggery, and coconut to a pan and sauté on low flame until cooked.
2. Add the milk and cook until the mixture is dry. Let it cool.
3. Add milk powder.
4. Roll into *laddoos*.
5. Spread the sesame seeds on a plate. Roll the *laddoos* in the seeds so they are covered.

Porridge

This porridge is easily digestible, takes 5 minutes to prepare, and can form a complete meal when you need something light and nutritious. Ragi and *rajgeera* are alkaline foods and high in calcium. Soy is a good source of vegetable protein.

Ingredients

- 250 grams of ragi flour
- 100 grams of *rajgeera* flour
- 100 grams of soy flour
- 50 grams of dry date powder (*kharik* powder)
- 50 grams of almonds
- 10 grams of *methi* powder
- Ghee, water, salt, milk, and jaggery as required

Directions

1. Mix all the ingredients except ghee and store them in a container for use whenever you need.
2. To make one portion of porridge, take 1 tablespoon of the mixture and roast on low flame with 1tsp of ghee. Add water slowly and stir consistently. Add a pinch of salt. Add milk and jaggery if you want them.

Brownie Balls

Ingredients

- ½ cup of walnuts
- ½ cup of almonds
- 1 cup of large dates, chopped
- 1/3 cup + 2 teaspoons of unsweetened cocoa powder
- ½ cup of shredded coconut flakes
- pinch of salt

Directions

1. Grind the walnuts and almonds in a food processor until a dough starts to form.
2. Add the dates, 1/3 cup of cocoa powder, ¼ cup of shredded coconut flakes and salt and process until incorporated and the mixture begins to turn into a dough.
3. Roll the mixture into round balls.
4. Mix the remaining ¼ cup shredded coconut flakes and 2 teaspoons cocoa and roll the balls in this mixture.
5. Place in the fridge for at least an hour, then enjoy!

Miscellaneous

Vegetable Broth

This broth is full of nutrients and can serve as a soup in itself. If you are unable to eat solids or need to eat every few hours, this is a great option. You can experiment with its taste by adding or eliminating the spices you like. Ginger, cloves, and cinnamon are options. If celery or parsley are not easily available, just omit them. If you want a clear broth, leave out the tomatoes.

Ingredients

- ½ kg of onions, cut into large pieces
- ½ kg of carrots, cut into 1-inch pieces
- ½ kg of tomatoes, cored
- ½ kg of green capsicum
- ¼ kg of radish
- 2 tablespoons of cold pressed oil or any other unrefined oil
- 3 cloves of garlic
- 3 whole cloves
- 1 bay leaf
- 6 whole black peppercorns
- 1 bunch of fresh coriander leaves, chopped
- 3.5 liters of water

Directions

1. Heat 1 tsp of oil in a flat pan. Slowly cook onions, carrots, tomatoes, bell peppers, and radish over a low flame, tossing every two minutes until nicely cooked.
2. Put the browned vegetables, celery, garlic, cloves, bay leaf, pepper corns, Italian parsley, and water into a large stock pot. Bring to a full boil. Reduce heat to simmer. Cook uncovered until liquid is reduced by half.
3. Pour the broth through a colander, catching the broth in a large bowl or pot. This liquid is your vegetable broth, and it can be used immediately or stored for later. It will last in your fridge for three days. You can also freeze the broth in ice cube trays for easy use. The strained vegetables are delicious since they have absorbed all the flavor of the spices. You can eat them hot or cold.

Homemade Porridge Powder

Ingredients

- 1 cup of rice
- 1 cup of *moong* dal
- 4 tbsp of red *masoor* dal
- 2 tbsp of almonds

Directions

1. Mix all ingredients and rinse well with water. Drain and dry on a cotton cloth.
2. Place in a pan and roast on slow flame.
3. Grind into powder and store in a steel container in the refrigerator. Stays fresh for about 6 weeks.
4. To use: Mix 2 tbsps. of powder in ½ cup of water. Boil 1 cup of water. Add the above mixture, stir, and cook. Do not add sugar. You may add a pinch of salt. In about 5 minutes, the porridge will be ready. You may enhance the flavor with a spoonful of pure ghee.

Soya Chunks Recipe

Ingredients

- 1 cup of soybeans
- 1 tsp of coriander powder
- 1 tsp of cumin
- ¼ tsp of asafetida
- ½ tsp of chili powder
- salt to taste

Directions

1. Soak beans overnight. Drain water and grind with all the spices.
2. Make small chunks of the mixture on a plastic sheet and leave for 2 days to dry in the sun. If natural sunlight is not available, then you can dry roast or bake. Ensure that there is no moisture left, otherwise the chunks become stale and moldy.
3. Store in a dry container.

Homemade Ketchup

Store-bought ketchup and tomato sauces have loads of sugar, chemicals, and preservatives. If you use ketchup regularly, then you should make your own.

Ingredients

- 1 kilo of tomatoes, cooked and pureed
- ½ cup of water, divided
- 2/3 cup of white sugar
- ¾ cup of distilled white vinegar
- 1 teaspoon of onion powder
- 1/2 teaspoon of garlic powder
- 1 and ¾ teaspoons of salt
- 1/8 teaspoon of mustard powder
- ¼ teaspoon of finely ground black pepper
- 1 whole clove
- ¼ teaspoon chili powder

Directions

1. Pour ground tomatoes into a slow cooker. Swirl ½ cup of water.
2. Add sugar, vinegar, onion powder, garlic powder, salt, mustard powder, black pepper, chili powder and whole clove; whisk to combine.
3. Cook uncovered on high, until the mixture is reduced by half and very thick (4-5 hours). Stir every hour or so.
4. Smooth the texture of the ketchup using a blender for about 20 seconds.
5. Put mixture through a fine strainer to take skins and seeds out.
6. Transfer the strained ketchup to a bowl.
7. Cool completely before tasting to adjust salt, black pepper, or cayenne pepper.

Protein Powder with Omega-3s (No Preservatives)

This homemade mixture has no preservatives and can be used in chutneys, salads, *sabjis*, dals, and other prepared foods to increase its protein and omega-3 content. It can be added to wheat flour, dal, pancakes, khichdi, and cooked rice to increase the protein value of foods and to provide daily natural omega. This powder is rich in natural calcium and each 10-gram serving provides 4 grams of protein.

Ingredients

- Peanuts 100 gms.
- Roasted Chana Dal (called chivada-dal or futana dal) 100 gms
- Watermelom seeds 100 gms
- Pumpkin seeds 100 gms
- Walnuts 50 gms
- Cashews 50 gms
- Almonds 50 gms
- Sesame seeds 50 gms
- Watermelon seeds 50 gms
- Chia seeds 50 gms
- Flaxseeds 100 gms
- (Total 700gm)

Directions

1. Roast peanuts and remove the skin.
2. Roast all other seeds and nuts on medium flame.
3. Grind carefully to make a fine powder. Do not over-grind, as this will cause releasing of oil.
4. Store in a glass/steel container once cooled.
5. This mixture keeps for 15-20 days if stored in a glass/steel container.

Cancer Protective Omega-3 Badishep

Ingredients

- 200 grams of *badishep* (fennel seeds)
- 50 grams of *dhana* dal
- 25 grams of *ajwain* seeds
- 25 grams of flaxseeds
- 10 grams of sesame seeds
- 10 grams of chia seeds
- 25 grams of walnut pieces
- 10 grams of watermelon seeds

Directions

1. Roast ingredients separately.
2. Mix and store.
3. Have a teaspoon after meals.

Homemade Mouthwashes

Homemade Mouthwash 1

Ingredients

- 300 ml of filtered water
- 2 tsp of cloves
- 1 tsp of ground cinnamon
- 1 tsp of peppermint oil or any other flavoring you may like (vanilla, almond or lavender)

Directions

1. Boil water with the cinnamon and cloves until the water has boiled and decreased by half. Let it cool for 20 minutes.
2. Strain the liquid in a fine-meshed strainer.
3. Add the flavoring and store it in a glass bottle.

Homemade Mouthwash 2

Ingredients

- 1 cup of aloe vera juice
- 1 cup of water
- 2 tsp of baking soda
- ¼ tsp of rock salt (*kala namak*)

Directions

1. Mix and store in the fridge.
2. Shake before using.

Homemade Mouthwash 3

Ingredients

- ½ inch of grated ginger
- 10-15 coarsely chopped mint leaves
- 1 tsp of turmeric
- 1 tsp of cinnamon
- 3 cups of water

Directions

1. Simmer all the ingredients over a low flame for about half an hour.
2. Cool, strain, and store in the fridge.
3. Shake before using.

Anti-Cancer Regional Dishes

Volumes of recipes books would not be enough to encapsulate all of India's recipes. Each state, each village, each community, and each home have their own unique cuisine. There are a countless number of healthy traditional food preparations, and it was difficult to narrow them down. This list by state, showcases the diversity of our food culture. We do not include the actual recipes because there are numerous ways to make the same dish and so many versions of them are readily available online.

1. Andhra Pradesh

Panasa Putty Koora (jackfruit curry)

- **Why We Chose It:** This delicious curry is made of fresh coconut and cashew. Raw jackfruit is marinated with various healthy spices, mostly mustard seeds. Proteins from lentils and antioxidants from jackfruit makes this a wholesome and healthy dish.
- **Cancer Protective Elements:** jackfruit, nuts, spices, lentils

2. Arunachal Pradesh

Zan (finger millet porridge with vegetables)

- **Why We Chose It:** This tribal recipe is high in fiber, very satisfying with almost no oil or ghee. Basic modes of cooking like steaming and boiling make this dish easily digestible and economical.

- **Cancer Protective Elements:** finger millet (ragi), carrot, spinach, soya beans, green peas coriander
- **Suggestions:** In Urban areas, modified versions of this dish use ghee to fry the ragi flour first. In some recipes cheese is also used. Try and stick to the traditional mode of cooking.

3. Assam

Papaya Khaar (raw papaya with lentils)

- **Why We Chose It:** *Khaar* is made by charring dried banana peels and grinding to a fine powder. This ash is stored in water and used in various Assamese dishes. The ash water gives an alkaline edge to the food. It is also gut friendly.
- **Cancer Protective Elements:** Lentils, raw papaya, spices, herbs, *khaar*.

   Note: In the present day instead of traditional *khaar*, baking soda is used in the same recipes and the good effects of *khaar* are no longer in the dish.

4. Bihar

Sattu Sherbat

- **Why We Chose It:** This energy booster drink will win you over with the simplicity of its ingredients. It may be the only sherbet in the country that uses no sugar or jaggery.
- **Cancer Protective Elements:** roasted chickpeas, spices, mint, onion

5. Chattisgarh

Kandbhaji (sweet potato leaf curry)

- **Why We Chose It:** Chattisgarh, the rice bowl of India, has a rich traditional cuisine and has on its land over 50 types of leafy vegetables. *Kandbhaji* is one of them. Sweet potato leaves are rich in beta carotene, various antioxidants and minerals. Lentils give it a protein edge.

- **Cancer Protective Elements:** leafy greens, tomato, garlic, onion, lentils

6. Goa
Muddoyshya Hooman (lady fish curry)

- **Why We Chose It:** This dish has the goodness of coconut, lady fish and turmeric.
- **Cancer Protective Elements:** Lady fish has high levels of omega-3 fatty acids, proteins, iodine, and vitamin D.

7. Gujrat
Handvo (savory lentil cake)

- **Why We Chose It:** Handvo is rich in all macronutrients (carbs, proteins and fats). A combination of prebiotic and probiotic foods make it beneficial for gut health and being a fermented dish, the proteins are well absorbed. It is also a good dish for weight gain.
- **Cancer Protective Elements:** Lentils, herbs, carrot, seeds, and spices
- **Suggestions:** You can use cabbage in place of bottle gourd for an anti-cancer edge. Load up all types of veggies for variety.

8. Hariyana
Bajra Khichdi (pearl millet savory porridge)

- **Why We Chose It:** This dish is high in iron and good for diabetics with its low glycemic index.
- Cancer protective elements: millets and spices
- Suggestions: Have this *khichdi* with *kadhi* or *raita*.

9. Himachal Pradesh

Siddhu (dimsums/momos)

- **Why We Chose It:** Use of walnut, rajma, and poppy seeds makes this Pahadi dish extremely nutritious and anti-cancer.
- **Cancer Protective Elements:** walnuts, poppy seeds, herbs and spices
- **Suggestions:** Traditionally *patal* (leaves) were used to wrap the *siddhu*. Now with the momo steamer wrapping with leaves is rarely used. However, you can use locally available leaves for added flavor. It is traditionally eaten with green chutney. Do not eat with ketchup or sauce.

10. Jharkhand

Rugra (rugda mushroom)

- **Why We Chose It:** The *rugda* mushroom is indigenous to the state of Jharkhand. It is considered to be anti-diabetic and anti-cancer.
- **Cancer Protective Elements:** *rugda* mushrooms

11. Karnataka

Bisi Bele Bath (hot lentil rice)

- **Why We Chose It:** This one- pot dish uses super healthy components like fenugreek seeds, coriander seeds, cinnamon, cloves and more. The dish is a complete protein and has the goodness of vegetables.
- **Cancer protective elements:** carrots, capsicum, french beans, green peas, spices, lentils

12. Kashmir

Kahwa (green tea)

- **Why We Chose It:** It is a soulful drink rich in vitamins. If this is taken after meals it has a fat burning effect due to raised metabolism.
- **Cancer protective elements:** green tea, saffron, nuts

13. Kerala
Vegetable Isthu (vegetable stew)
- **Why We Chose It:** *Isthu* is cooked in coconut oil which is considered one the best fat choices and the sumptuous use of a variety of vegetables, spices, and herbs makes this dish quite potent on the health scale. The coconut milk used is good dietary tool for weight gain, making the dish best for those suffering from weight loss.
- **Cancer Protective Elements:** Carrots, beans, spices, coconut
- **Suggestions:** If you are worried about the calories, you can use grated coconut instead of coconut milk, this will maintain the taste and include added fiber. Do not limit yourself to specific vegetables, use a variety including sweet potato, cauliflower, etc.

14. Madhya Pradesh
Chakke ki Saag, Dal Bafla
- **Why We Chose It:** This dish is similar to Rajasthan's famous *dal baati* or Bihar's *litti*. Copious use of whole grains and lentils makes it a complete balanced meal.
- **Cancer protective elements:** whole grains, lentils, turmeric
- **Suggestions:** Go easy on the ghee

15. Maharashtra
Thalipith (savory pancake)
- **Why We Chose It:** This nutritious dish is ideal for today's lifestyle. It is high in protein, rich in vitamins, minerals, fiber and antioxidants.
- **Cancer protective elements:** millets, wholegrains, lentils, spices, seeds
- **Suggestions:** Add grated cabbage, leafy greens, moringa powder for a greater nutritional advantage. Do not have it with ketchup or sauce. Any dry chutney and *dahi* will go well with it.

16. Manipur

- *Eromba* (stew with fermented bamboo shoots)
- **Why We Chose It:** It is rich in fiber and anti-inflammatory foods. Fermented dried fish makes this dish unique.
- Cancer Protective Elements – fermented bamboo shoots, buckwheat, yam stem, eisholtzia blanda leaves (mint family).

17. Meghalaya

Bamboo Shoot Curry

- **Why We Chose It:** This gem of a dish uses locally available bamboo shoots which have anti-cancer properties. If traditionally prepared it requires no oil.
- **Cancer protective elements:** bamboo shoots
- **Suggestions:** If you are vegetarian you may replace fermented fish with lentils.

18. Mizoram

Chhum Han (steamed vegetables)

- **Why We Chose It:** This simple dish makes use of cruciferous vegetables which have potent anti-cancer properties.
- Cancer Protective Elements: carrot, cabbage, broccoli, cauliflower.
- Suggestions: Do not add butter, do not overcook vegetables.

19. Nagaland

Hinkejvu (boiled vegetables)

- **Why We Chose It:** This potent dish is rich in leafy vegetables, root vegetables, and beans. There is no oil used and it is high in prebiotics.
- **Cancer Protective Elements:** colocasia root, cabbage, mustard leaves, green beans.

20. Orissa
Dalma (lentils cooked with vegetables)

- **Why We Chose It:** This traditional dish is power packed with antioxidants and phytochemicals. In Orissa a healthy spice mixture called "pancha phutana" is used to temper many dishes. The mixture is a combination of cumin, mustard, fennel, fenugreek and black cumin seeds. Veggies like brinjals, raw papaya, beans, etc. give a healthy edge to this dish.
- **Cancer Protective Elements:** brinjals, raw papaya, beans, carrots, lentils, spices.

21. Punjab
Sarson ka Saag (mustard leaves vegetable)

- **Why We Chose It:** This dish is rich in 3 types of green leafy vegetables – mustard greens, spinach and *bathua*. There is traditionally quite a bit of butter in this recipe but if it is omitted or reduced this *saag* becomes a superb weight loss dish with power packed nutrition.
- **Cancer protective elements:** leafy greens, herbs and spices
- **Suggestions:** You can add proteins to the saag by adding chickpea flour instead of corn flour. Traditionally this is had with *Makka ki Roti* (corn roti). Also, go easy on the butter while serving.

22. Rajasthan
Gatte ki Sabji (chickpea flour dumpling)

- **Why Why We Chose It:** This nostalgic meal from Rajasthan is cooked in a variety of ways. It's high protein content and richness of spices makes it a wholesome dish.
- **Cancer protective elements:** lentils, spices, herbs
- **Suggestions:** Go easy on the ghee.

23. Sikkim
Gundruk (fermented dried leafy greens)
- **Why We Chose It:** This Nepalese origin dish gives probiotic as well as prebiotic benefits. It can be added to soups and other vegetable dishes.
- **Cancer Protective Elements:** cabbage leaves, mustard leaves, radish leaves.

24. Tamil Nadu
Idli Sambar
- **Why We Chose It:** Although native to Tamil Nadu this wonderful dish is available all over India. The fermentation procedure of the *idli* makes it rich in proteins and gut friendly. The high protein sambar can accommodate all sorts of different vegetables without losing its flavor. This dish is low in fat and very satisfying.
- **Cancer Protective Elements:** lentils, spices, herbs, and vegetables like drumsticks, pumpkin, etc.

25. Telangana
Qubani ka Meetha
- **Why We Chose It:** We chose this because the dried apricots in this dish have anti-oxidant properties which help neutralize cancer causing free radicals. The use of saffron, almonds, and cardamom helps enhance not just the flavor but the nutritive value as well.
- **Suggestions:** Skip adding cream. The dish is tasty on its own and there is no need to increase the fat content.

26. Tripura
Panch Phoran Tarkari (mixed vegetable dish)
- **Why We Chose It:** This Bengali inspired dish is full of alkaline

vegetables and uses a combination of 5 healthy spices called *panch phoran* – cumin seeds, nigella seeds, wild celery seeds (*radhuni*), fenugreek seeds and fennel seeds.

- **Cancer protective elements:** pumpkin, brinjal, *panch phoran* spices

27. Uttarakhand
Lingude Ki Sabji (fiddle head fern)

- **Why We Chose It:** This "Pahadi" dish is also well known by other names in other states. It is *dhekia* in Assam, *dheli saag* in Tripura and *kasrod* in Kashmir. This asparagus-like plant is super rich in vitamins and minerals and most importantly fiber.
- **Cancer protective elements:** carotenoids, prebiotics and organic as it is a naturally grown plant in jungles

28. Uttar Pradesh
Chauli Saag (amaranth leaves sabji)

- **Why We Chose It:** Amaranth leaves are a very alkaline green leafy vegetable rich in antioxidants and fiber.
- **Cancer protective elements:** amaranth leaves, garlic, onion, tomato
- **Suggestions:** You can mix spinach with the *chauli*, as is done in some villages, making it more nutritious.

29. West Bengal
Shukto (mixed vegetable dish)

- **Why We Chose It:** This nutritious dish is a treasure trove of anti-cancer vegetables. The use of the Bengali spice "*radhuri*" makes it more unique. *Radhuri* which is dried celery is a dried fruit of a plant which has anti-cancer properties.
- **Cancer protective elements:** drumsticks, bitter gourd, radish, brinjal, raw banana ridge gourd, red pumpkin, wild celery seeds

- **Suggestions:** Traditionally some vegetables are deep fried. This does add calories but the oil helps in absorption of certain nutrients, so making it the traditional way is okay.

> *Do you agree with our choices of cancer protective dishes from your native region? If you have any other suggestions, please mail your thoughts to us. We would love to know more about the rich regional cuisine of our country.*
> *Email us at: changingthewayindiaeats@gmail.com*

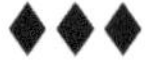

References

- Arnold, M. *et al.* (2016) *Obesity and cancer: An update of the global impact, Cancer Epidemiology*. Available at: https://www.sciencedirect.com/science/article/abs/pii/S1877782116000059
- Bhatia, Dr. Arti (2018) *Cancer, Your Body and Your Diet: A Vital Journey*. New Delhi: Speaking Tiger Publishing Pvt. Ltd.
- Bhide, M. (2011) *The crackling spices of Indian tempering, NPR*. Available at: https://www.npr.org/2011/12/07/143251451/the-crackling-spices-of-indian-tempering
- Charaka. *Charaka Samhita*
- Dia, V.P. and Krishnan, H.B. (2016) 'BG-4, a novel anticancer peptide from bitter gourd (momordica charantia), promotes apoptosis in human colon cancer cells', *Scientific Reports*, 6(1). doi:10.1038/srep33532.
- Eslami, M. *et al.* (2019) 'Importance of probiotics in the prevention and treatment of colorectal cancer', *Journal of Cellular Physiology*, 234(10), pp. 17127–17143. doi:10.1002/jcp.28473.
- *Gheranda Samhita.*
- Ghosh, Dr. A. (2016) 'Coconut: Natural source of potential anti cancer agent', *CORD*, 32(1), p. 9. doi:10.37833/cord.v32i1.45.
- Hajare, R. (2017) 'Milk fact not fiction it has contrast medicine:

Revise', *Advances in Complementary & Alternative Medicine*, 1(1). doi:10.31031/acam.2017.01.000503.

- Isaksen, I.M. and Dankel, S.N. (2023) 'Ultra-processed food consumption and cancer risk: A systematic review and meta-analysis', *Clinical Nutrition*, 42(6), pp. 919–928. doi:10.1016/j.clnu.2023.03.018.

- Kajale, M.D. (1974) 'Ancient Grains From India', *Bulletin of the Deccan College Post-Graduate and Research Institute*, 34(1/4), pp. 55–74. Available at: https://www.jstor.org/stable/42931019.

- Katzin, C. (2018) *The Cancer Nutrition Center Handbook*. Fountain Resources

- Keane, M. and Chace, D. (2007) *What to eat if you have cancer: Healing Foods that boost your immune system*. New York: McGraw-Hill.

- Kour, Harminder (2017) 'Evaluation of In Vitro Anticancer Potential of Some Vegetables From Jammu Region', *Sher-e-Kashmir*, University of Agricultural Sciences nd Technology of Jammu.

- Lappano, R. *et al.* (2017) 'The lauric acid-activated signaling prompts apoptosis in cancer cells', *Cell Death Discovery*, 3(1). doi:10.1038/cddiscovery.2017.63.

- Lee, S.-H. *et al.* (2020) 'Emotional well-being and gut microbiome profiles by enterotype', *Scientific Reports*, 10(1). doi:10.1038/s41598-020-77673-z.

- Limaye, Dr. Arvind (2012) *Annapuran*. Mehta Publishing

- Longvah, T., Ananthan, R., Bhaskarachary, K., Venkaiah, K. (2017) *Indian Food Composition Tables*. Hyderabad: National Institute of Nutrition.

- Mohamad, N.E. *et al.* (2019) 'In vitro and in vivo antitumour effects of coconut water vinegar on 4t1 breast cancer cells', *Food & Nutrition Research*, 63(0). doi:10.29219/fnr.v63.1616.

- National Cancer Institute (2018) *Eating Hints: Before, During &*

After Cancer Treatment. Independently published.

- Prasad, K.N. & Prasad, K.C. (2011) *Fighting Cancer With Vitamins and Antioxidants.* Healing Arts Press.

- Prerna, S. *et al.* (2022) 'In Vitro and In Vivo Anticancer Activity of Basil (*Ocimum* spp.): Current Insights and Future Prospects', *Cancers (Basel)* 14(10):2375. doi: 10.3390/cancers14102375.

- Purwal, L. *et al.* (2010) 'In vivo anticancer activity of the leaves and fruits of Moringa oleifera on mouse melanoma', *Pharmacology Online* 1:655-656.

- Sarwate, Dr. Nandini (2016) *Dietary Advice for Cancer Patients.* Mumbai: JASCAP.

- Sharma, V. *et al.* (2021) 'Probiotics and prebiotics having broad spectrum anticancer therapeutic potential: Recent trends and future perspectives', *Current Pharmacology Reports*, 7(2), pp. 67–79. doi:10.1007/s40495-021-00252-x.

- Shoba, G. *et al.* (1997) 'Influence of piperine on the pharmacokinetics of curcumin in animals and human volunteers', *Planta Medica*, 64(04), pp. 353–356. doi:10.1055/s-2006-957450.

- Svatmarama. *Hathpradipika.*

- Vagbhata. *Ashtangasangraha.*

- Vagbhata. *Ashtangahridayam.*

- Wei, D. *et al.* (2018) 'Probiotics for the prevention or treatment of chemotherapy- or radiotherapy-related diarrhoea in people with cancer', *Cochrane Database of Systematic Reviews*, 2018(8). doi:10.1002/14651858.cd008831.pub3.